DIET, NUTRITION, AND CANCER: FROM BASIC RESEARCH TO POLICY IMPLICATIONS

CURRENT TOPICS IN NUTRITION AND DISEASE

Series Editors
 Anthony A. Albanese
 The Burke Rehabilitation Center
 White Plains, New York

 David Kritchevsky
 The Wistar Institute
 Philadelphia, Pennsylvania

DIET, NUTRITION, AND CANCER: FROM BASIC RESEARCH TO POLICY IMPLICATIONS

Proceedings of a Workshop Held at Cornell University
Ithaca, New York
August 1982

Editor

Daphne A. Roe, MD
Division of Nutritional Sciences
Cornell University
Ithaca, New York

Alan R. Liss, Inc., New York

Library of Congress Cataloging in Publication Data
Main entry under title:

Diet, nutrition, and cancer.

(Current topics in nutrition and disease; v. 9)
Bibliography: p.
Includes index.
1. Cancer—Nutritional aspects—Congresses.
2. Cancer—Prevention—Congresses. 3. Carcinogenesis—
Congresses. I. Roe, Daphne A. II. Series.
RC262.D515 1983   616.99'4   83-9909
ISBN 0-8451-1608-8

Contents

MUTAGENS AND CANCER

RISK ASSESSMENT: EXPERIMENTAL AND EPIDEMIOLOGICAL

PUBLIC POLICY

Contributors

Leonard F. Bjeldanes, Department of Nutritional Sciences, University of California, Berkeley, CA 94720 **[177]**

Homer S. Black, Photobiology Laboratory, Veterans Administration Medical Center, and Department of Dermatology, Baylor College of Medicine, Houston, TX 77211 **[49]**

Colin Campbell, Division of Nutritional Sciences, Cornell University, Ithaca, NY 14853 **[1]**

Margaret C. Cheney, Department of National Health and Welfare, Health Protection Building, Tunney's Pasture, Ottawa, Ontario, Canada K1A 0L2 **[257]**

Frank Chytil, Department of Biochemistry, Vanderbilt University School of Medicine, Nashville, TN 37232 **[117]**

Luigi M. De Luca, Differentiation Control Section, National Cancer Institute, Bethesda, MD 20205 **[111]**

James S. Felton, Biomedical Sciences Division, Livermore National Laboratory, University of California, Livermore, CA 94550 **[177]**

Allan L. Forbes, Office of the Associate Director for Nutrition and Food Sciences, Bureau of Foods, Food and Drug Administration, Washington, DC 20204 **[269]**

Mary Y. Fukayama, Department of Environmental Toxicology, University of California at Davis, Davis, CA 95616 **[155]**

Frederick T. Hatch, Biomedical Sciences Division, Lawrence Livermore National Laboratory, University of California, Livermore, CA 94550 **[177]**

Dennis P.H. Hsieh, Department of Environmental Toxicology, University of California at Davis, Davis, CA 95616 **[155]**

M. Margaret King, Biomembrane Medical Research Foundation, Oklahoma Medical Research Foundation, Oklahoma City, OK 73104 **[61]**

Mark G. Knize, Biomedical Sciences Division, Lawrence Livermore National Laboratory, University of California, Livermore, CA 94550 **[177]**

Gene Liau, Department of Biochemistry, Vanderbilt University School of Medicine, Nashville, TN 37232 **[117]**

Daniel S. Longnecker, Department of Pathology, Dartmouth Medical School, Hanover, NH 03756 **[33]**

Joyce McCann, Biomedical Division, Lawrence Berkeley Laboratory, University of California, Berkeley, CA 94720 **[137]**

The number in brackets is the opening page number of the contributor's article.

Paul B. McCay, Biomembrane Research Laboratory, Oklahoma Medical Research Foundation, Oklahoma City, OK 73104 **[7,61]**

Gail McKeown-Eyssen, Ludwig Institute for Cancer Research, Toronto Branch, and University of Toronto, Toronto, Ontario, Canada M5S 1A1 **[243]**

Curtis Mettlin, Department of Cancer Control and Epidemiology, Roswell Park Memorial Institute, Buffalo, NY 14263 **[125]**

Masahide Omori, Department of Biochemistry, Vanderbilt University School of Medicine, Nashville, TN 37232 **[117]**

David E. Ong, Department of Biochemistry, Vanderbilt University School of Medicine, Nashville, TN 37232 **[117]**

Bandaru S. Reddy, Nutritional Biochemistry, American Health Foundation, Naylor Dana Institute for Disease Prevention, Valhalla, NY 10595 **[17]**

David W. Rice, Department of Environmental Toxicology, University of California at Davis, Davis, CA 95616 **[155]**

Daphne A. Roe, Division of Nutritional Sciences, Cornell University, Ithaca, NY 14853 **[ix]**

B.D. Roebuck, Department of Pharmacology and Toxicology, Dartmouth Medical School, Hanover, NH 03756 **[33]**

Miriam P. Rosin, Environmental Carcinogenesis Unit, British Columbia Cancer Research Centre, Vancouver, British Columbia, Canada V5Z 1L3 **[141]**

Irma H. Russo, Experimental Pathology Laboratory, Department of Biology, Michigan Cancer Foundation, Detroit, MI 48201 **[61]**

Marvin A. Schneiderman, Clement Associates, Inc., Arlington, VA **[221]**

David Schottenfeld, Epidemiology & Preventive Medicine Service, Memorial Sloan-Kettering Cancer Center, New York, NY 10021 **[197]**

Raymond E. Schucker, Office of the Associate Director for Nutrition and Food Sciences, Bureau of Foods, Food and Drug Administration, Washington, DC 20204 **[269]**

Patricia J. Steele, National Department of Health and Welfare, National Evaluation Division, Health Protection Building, Tunney's Pasture, Ottawa, Ontario, Canada K1A 0L2 **[257]**

Hans F. Stich, Environmental Carcinogenesis Unit, British Columbia Cancer Research Centre, Vancouver, British Columbia, Canada V5Z 1L3 **[141]**

Walter Troll, Environmental Medicine, New York University Medical Center, New York, NY 10016 **[167]**

John H. Weisburger, Naylor Dana Institute for Disease Prevention, American Health Foundation, Valhalla, NY 10595 **[203]**

Gary M. Williams, Experimental Pathology and Toxicology, Naylor Dana Institute for Disease Prevention, American Health Foundation, Valhalla, NY 10595 **[203]**

George Wolf, Department of Nutrition and Food Science, Massachusetts Institute of Technology, Cambridge, MA 02139 **[93]**

Jonathan Yavelow, Environmental Medicine, New York University Medical Center, New York, NY 10016 **[167]**

Stuart H. Yuspa, Laboratory of Cellular Carcinogenesis and Tumor Promotion, National Cancer Institute, Bethesda, MD 20205 **[95]**

Preface

The objective of this workshop was to enquire about mechanisms determining the carcinogenic and anticancer effects of nutrients as well as other food components. Our aim was also to evaluate the extent to which this information should be used in public regulatory programs.

Presently, any discussion of relationships between diet and cancer may lead to provocative debate. However, the hot debate of today may sometimes reflect the scientific progress of yesterday. The workshop "Diet, Nutrition, and Cancer: From Basic Research to Policy Implications" was innovative in that it provided a foundation for experimental oncologists and nutritionists to present their most recent studies of the role of nutrients and non-nutrients in food in carcinogenesis, and it also addressed the implications of laboratory research for the risk of human cancer and the possibility of cancer prevention.

We were extremely fortunate to get Paul McCay to chair the session on lipids, Joyce McCann to convene a group of papers on food mutagens and antimutagens, and George Wolf to chair a session on vitamin A and the retinoids. We were equally pleased to have David Schottenfeld bring an outstanding team together to discuss risk assessment and Sanford Miller to get speakers from regulatory agencies to consider policy decisions.

This book, in which the proceedings of the workshop are published, represents our effort to provide those who were unable to attend with new knowledge about diet and cancer and an awareness of how that knowledge may be interpreted and used in cancer prevention. All contributions to the workshop are included in this volume other than the Overview statements of Richard Peto and Sanford Miller. With these exceptions, the papers are grouped as they were presented.

As Editor of the Proceedings, I am deeply indebted to my colleague Colin Campbell, whose enthusiasm and genius brought this workshop to fruition. He chaired the organizing committee and selected the chairs of workshop sessions, coordinated the development of the workshop, and presided over the meeting.

I owe a special debt of thanks to Joan McLain and to Beverly Hastings, who gave invaluable secretarial assistance, and to Paulette Cohen of Alan R. Liss, Inc., who behind the scenes did so much of the work that made this publication possible.

I also wish to extend our deepest gratitude to those who contributed to the financial support of the meeting: American Petroleum Institute, Celanese Corporation, Coca-Cola Company, The Dow Chemical Company, Hoffmann-La Roche, Inc., M.E.D. Communications, M & M Mars, Pfizer Central Research, Quaker Oats Company, and Reed & Carnrick Pharmaceuticals. Without their generosity this workshop would not have taken place.

Daphne A. Roe, MD

Diet, Nutrition, and Cancer:
From Basic Research to Policy Implications, pages 1–4
© *1983 Alan R. Liss, Inc., 150 Fifth Avenue, New York, NY 10011*

OPENING REMARKS FOR WORKSHOP

Colin Campbell

Division of Nutritional Sciences
Cornell University
Ithaca, New York   14853

The principle objective of this workshop is "to inquire about the nature and mechanisms of the carcinogenic effects of nutrients and the extent to which this information could or should be used in public regulatory and educational programs."

For a workshop of this type, we are likely to be best served by limiting ourselves to the general observation derived from the literature which illustrates that a wide variety of nutrients are capable of modifying tumor development in a wide variety of tumor systems. In addition to this diversity of response, there is also impressive magnitude in some of these nutrient-induced effects, as well as concordance between human, animal and in vitro studies. Perhaps of most significance is the finding that nutrient-induced effects are oftentimes well within the range of traditional nutrient intakes. In a sense, that observation suggests that studies on nutrients may be more relevant than many of the studies on traditional chemical carcinogens, wherein experimental doses far beyond traditional exposure levels are oftentimes required. Is it therefore possible, particularly when nutrients are considered collectively, that their intakes may be major etiologic factors in the cancer process?

The implications of that hypothesis are rather enormous, it would seem. But, before these speculations are pushed too far, several questions need to be thoughtfully and carefully evaluated. How large and comprehensive are these effects? What is the relevance of primary, as opposed to interacting, nutrient effects? Are their experimentally derived mechanisms of action consistent with the human data base?

The first two sessions will address these questions, among others. The nutrients chosen for study - lipids and retinoids - were selected as case studies primarily because of their large bodies of literature. Moreover, they represent quite different nutrient classes insofar as intake manipulation is concerned. Lipid intake may be readily modified both by voluntary food selection and by food preparation, whereas retinoid or carotenoid intake could be altered both by food selection and by food fortification and/or supplementation. Paul McCay has organized a session focused on the question of breadth of action, as related to the lipid effect in diverse tumor model systems. This session will also consider the carcinogenesis phase most related to lipid intake, as well as lipid interactions with antioxidants, as a possible example of a nutrient-nutrient interaction. George Wolf will chair a session examining in some depth the mechanisms underlying retinoid activity in experimental animal and cell culture systems, concluding with a comparison of the cancer-related association of beta-carotene and preformed retinol intakes in humans.

If nutrient-induced effects on the cancer process are sufficiently significant, then how do they compare with tumor risks induced by classical chemical carcinogens which principally owe their activities to genotoxicity or mutagenicity? Historically, the correspondence between mutagenic and carcinogenic activities has been rather impressive, even though there are important aberrations. That is, there have been general implications that cancer risk may be related to the potencies and levels of exposure to mutagens. Prior to carcinogenicity testing, for example, candidate chemicals are submitted for initial screening to a battery of short-term tests. Considerable effort has been devoted to the determination of which test or battery of tests are most appropriate. Specific mechanisms and associative factors have been sought so that the aberrant responses might be better explained. That logic seemed in reasonably good order when Sugimura and his colleagues sprang a leak in that scheme when they discovered that compounds of extraordinary mutagenic potencies are being consumed at any time when food is cooked. The mutagenic potencies of

his amino acid pyrolysates make aflatoxin pale by comparison in the Salmonella TA98 system. Now we learn that
these compounds are also carcinogenic. Although their
potencies are less than predicted, a fair within-species
comparison with other carcinogens for diverse species has
not yet been obtained. What can be concluded? Should
cooking be prohibited? Hardly. Is it possible that in
most instances exposure to mutagens is already sufficiently diverse and comprised of sufficient potency to
permit the ultimate development of tumor response,
provided the other requisite etiologic factors are also
in order? Could nutrients be these other etiologic
factors? Joyce McCann has organized a comprehensive
session addressed to these and other questions. Perhaps
we can get some perspective by having these sessions on
nutrients and mutagens juxtaposed.

If nutrients prove to be sufficient tumor modifiers,
how can their intakes be assessed in terms of cancer
risk? Traditional dose-response risk assessment does not
seem appropriate. If nutrients primarily owe their
effects to the post-initiation phase, would that mean
that the parameters for time-to-tumor response become
more relevant? Because experimental nutrient intakes are
likely to be more relevant than chemical carcinogen
intakes, an evaluation of appropriate risk assessment
methodology for nutrients may be more rewarding than past
efforts addressed to high dose to low dose interpolation
and species to species extrapolation. Maybe with nutrients, epidemiological studies become more promising than
has been possible with traditional carcinogens. Dr.
Schottenfeld has organized a session addressed to questions concerning the role of epidemiological studies in
the assessment of nutrient activity.

And, finally, if nutrient action on the cancer
process should prove to be so significant as I've allowed
myself to imply, and methodology becomes available to
assess risk, then what public policy models are available
for the public arena? In the translation of such empiri-
cal data into public policy and marketplace activity,
what types of approaches are feasible? We should probably avoid straying into the philosophical question of
whether or not public policy making is legitimate on the
basis of information derived from this conference.
Current policy is already based on certain scientific
precepts and the real question is whether the new informa-

tion is sufficiently better than the old to lead to new policy. Let us simply assume that this information linking nutrition to cancer is sufficiently compelling at this time to warrant a preliminary discussion on what types of approaches would be useful to effect public policy, once the adequacy of the link is sufficiently established. Sandy Miller has acquired considerable experience in this type of activity and his session will offer presentations on a few selected concepts which should be considered.

LIPIDS AND CANCER

Diet, Nutrition, and Cancer:
From Basic Research to Policy Implications, pages 7–16
© *1983 Alan R. Liss, Inc., 150 Fifth Avenue, New York, NY 10011*

DIETARY FAT AND CANCER: AN OVERVIEW

Paul B. McCay, Ph.D.

Biomembrane Research Laboratory
Oklahoma Medical Research Foundation
Department of Biochemistry and Molecular Biology
University of Oklahoma Health Sciences Center
Oklahoma City, OK   73104

In 1930, Watson and Mellanby reported that dietary
fat modifies the response of animals to the tumorigenic
action of certain carcinogens (Watson, Mellanby 1930).
Later studies by Tannenbaum (Tannenbaum 1942).   Elevated
levels of dietary fat was later observed to be associated
with a significantly higher incidence of certain tumors in
response to carcinogens (Carroll, Khor 1970). Animals fed
high fat diets have also been observed to form greater
numbers of large tumors and metastatic lesions than did
animals given the same level of carcinogen but fed low
amounts of fat (Nigro, Singh, Campbell, Pak 1975). High
dietary fat levels have been reported to enhance the carcinogenic action of substances causing tumors in mammary
gland, liver, pancreas, small intestine, large intestine
and skin.

Tannenbaum has observed that the incidence of spontaneous mammary gland tumor in a strain of mice fed a diet
containing 28% fat was twice that of those fed the same
diet adjusted to contain 3% fat even though the animals
had not been exposed to any known carcinogen (Tannenbaum
1942). Furthermore, Carroll and coworkers have reported
that fat which contains higher amounts of unsaturated
fatty acids enhances carcinogen-induced tumor formation
and growth more effectively than fat containing high
levels of saturated fatty acids when fed at the same
caloric level (Gammal, Carrol, Plunkett 1967). Feeding
unsaturated fats increases the unsaturated fat content of

animal tissues, but whether or not this has significance
for the effect of dietary fat on chemical carcinogenesis
is not known. The studies of Carroll and Khor are consistent with the hypothesis that dietary fat (particularly
unsaturated fat) is a promoter of tumorigenesis by certain
chemical agents since the incidence is affected only by
the level or type of dietary fat fed after carcinogen
administration but not by the level or type of dietary fat
being consumed up to the time of carcinogen administration
(Carroll, Khor 1971). Since high levels of dietary fat
has a permissive action on the induction of the mixed-
function oxidase system, and since induction of this complex can enhance tumorigenesis when the induction is
carried out after administration of the carcinogen, it
appears possible that the effect of dietary fat on chemical carcinogenesis by compounds requiring metabolic activation may be mediated through its effect on this enzyme
complex.

The response of the drug metabolizing system to
dietary fat must be very complex. Hietanen et al. have
shown that hepatic microsomal aryl hydrocarbon hydroxylase
activity decreased markedly when rats were fed a diet
containing cocoa butter (control animals were fed a
standard rat ration) while the O-demethylase activity in
the same microsomal particles remained unchanged
(Hietanen, Laitinen, Vanio, Hanninen 1974). These investigators suggest that the fat may be affecting different
cytochrome P-450 species; P-450 in the case of the O-
demethylase and P_1-450 or P-448 in the case of the aryl
hydroxylase. It is clear that diets rich in lipids can
change the lipid composition of microsomes in various
organs, including the liver and the intestine, and this
could possibly affect the activity of various enzymic
components.

The evidence linking the metabolism of chemical carcinogens to the ultimate production of tumors is substantial, i.e., activation and conversion of polycyclic aromatic hydrocarbons, aromatic amines, and other compounds to
form products which ultimately interact with critical cell
components appears to be required for the transformation
of certain cell types to the neoplastic state. The conceptual aspects and much of the work supporting this
approach to the mechanism of the carcinogenesis was due to
the efforts of Miller and Miller (Miller, Miller 1969;

Miller 1971). Some exceptions to the activation requirement appear to be compounds which are effective alkylating
agents and some reactive nitrosamides. Yet even tumorigenesis by these compounds is enhanced by dietary fat.

The enzyme complex that appears to be the most critical in the metabolism of carcinogens to the activated or
ultimate form is the mixed-function oxidase system. This
system is present in many tissues in which the carcinogens
induce tumors. Mixed-function oxidase systems are present
in mammalian liver, including human liver (Levin, Conney,
Alvares 1972), and in other mammalian organs, including
kidney, lung, digestive tract (Nebert, Gelboin 1969);
adrenals (Omura, Sato, Cooper, Rosenthal, Estabrook 1965);
placenta (Nebert, Winker, Gelboin 1969); lymphocytes
(Whitlock, Cooper, Gelboin 1972); and monocytes (Bast,
Whitlock, Miller, Rapp, Gelboin 1974). The mixed-function
oxidase system is associated with the endoplasmic reticulum of those cells which contain the system. This oxidase
system in liver microsomes includes a reductase (NADPH-
cytochrome P-450 reductase) and cytochrome P-450. The
latter is now known to exist in multiple forms, several of
which can be distinguished by their specific properties
(Huang, West, Lu 1976; Guengerich 1977). The various
forms of cytochrome P-450 present in microsomes differ in
one or more of the following ways: molecular weight,
wavelength absorption maximum either in the oxidized state
or in the reduced state complexed to carbon monoxide,
substrate specificity, and response to inducing agents.
Some of the cytochromes can be distinguished by their
electrophoretic behavior (Atlas, Boobis, Felton,
Thorgeirsson, Nebert 1977). In addition to these
variables, there is also evidence that various tissues in
the same animals contain inducible cytochrome P-450-depen-
dent monoxygenase systems which have a different profile
of P-450 cytochromes and which respond differently to the
same inducing agents, indicating that separate genes must
be involved in the induction process. It appears likely
that the profiles of cytochrome P-450 vary from tissue to
tissue in the same animal. Furthermore, the age of the
animal appears to be a factor in determining the behavior
of the mixed-function oxidase system as well, since
monoxygenase activities which are present in very young
animals are found not to be present in the adults (Atlas,
Boobis, Felton, Thorgeirsson, Nebert 1977).

There is good evidence that dietary factors have a significant influence on monoxygenase systems in animal tissues. Many of these studies relate to the effect of nutritional deficiences on monoxygenase activity. Deficiencies of protein (Campbell, Hayes 1976), and certain vitamins (Newberne, Rogers 1973; Zannoni, Sato 1976) result in impaired activity. A deficiency of iron results in a significantly increased activity, while a deficiency of magnesium resulted in a lowering of capacity to metabolize various drugs (Becking 1976). The effect of the type and amount of dietary fat has a marked influence on the activity of the mixed-function oxidase systems in female rat liver. The rate (Vmax) of metabolism of different substrates is altered by dietary fat. Female rats fed a fat-free diet metabolize hexobarbital at only half the rate as do female rats fed a diet containing 3% corn oil, but aniline hydroxylation was unchanged (Norred, Wade 1972). It seems very likely that the drug metabolizing systems will be found to mediate the effects of dietary components in at least some tumor models.

The carcinogenic effect of 7,12-dimethylbenz(α)-anthracene (DMBA) is significantly enhanced when the level of corn oil was raised from 0.5% to 20% in a purified diet fed to female rats (Chan and Cohen 1974). Mammary tumors appeared earlier and in greater numbers than in rats fed the low-fat diet. Chan and Cohen also noted that an anti-estrogenic drug decreased DMBA-induced tumor incidence in both dietary groups but the high-fat diet group still exhibited higher incidence (Chan, Cohen 1974). On the other hand, an antiprolactin drug depressed the incidence of DMBA-induced mammary tumors and also abolished the difference in tumor incidence between the two dietary groups (Chan, Cohen 1974). This led these investigators to hypothesize that rats fed high fat levels in the diet secrete higher levels of prolactin than those fed low-fat diets. Their results correlated with those of Dunning et al. (Dunning, Curtis, Maun 1949) in which histological examination of the mammary gland in rats fed high-fat diets showed evidence of glandular hypertrophy and greater secretory activity. Reddy and coworkers have shown that a high fat-containing diet also enhanced the occurrence of tumors in the intestines of rats treated with dimethyl-hydrazine (Reddy, Weisberger, Wynder 1974). One hypothesis proposed is that enhancement of colon carcinogenesis by fat is related to metabolic conversion of bile acids by anaerobic bacteria in the intestine to substances which promote carcinogenesis (Aries, Crowther, Drasar, Hill, Williams 1969). Reddy and coworkers have shown that an increased secretion of bile acids into the intestinal tract caused by high levels of dietary fat might augment such conversion. However, the effect of elevated dietary fat levels on carcinogenesis in some tissues appears to involve other factors when additional facts are taken into consideration. First, although dimethylhydrazine-induced tumor formation in the intestine was enhanced, Rodgers and Newberne demonstrated that the incidence of tumors of the ear duct was depressed in rats fed a high fat diet which was marginally deficient in lipotropes (Rodgers, Newberne 1973). This would be difficult to explain on the basis of the production of a promoting agent in the intestine by anaerobic bacteria. Secondly, oxidized fats exhibit greater carcinogenic activity than fresh ones (Roffo 1946) suggesting that oxidized oils may contain tumor-promoting materials. This possible action of oxidized fat is supported by the studies of Sugai et al. (Sugai, Witting, Tsuchujama, Kummerow 1962), who demonstrated that diets containing heated vegetable oils increased the carcinogenicity of 2-acetylaminofluorene (AAF) in rats, causing a markedly greater incidence of mammary tumors in the mammary gland even in male rats. AAF ordinarily produces a preponderance of liver tumors in male rats. These workers suggested that lipid peroxides might react with AAF to form N-hydroxy-AAF which is a more potent carcinogen than AAF (Miller, Miller, Hartman 1961). Oxidized fat is known to contain hydroperoxides and epoxides (Artman 1969) among the various products formed.

The enhancement by dietary fat of the incidence of many types of carcinogen-induced tumors as well as spontaneously occurring neoplasms is now well-established and subject to experimental investigation as this morning's session will make apparent. The levels of dietary fat which cause significantly higher tumor yields in animal studies is well below the average per capita fat intake for the United States. Therefore, the possibility exists that many individuals with an inherited or acquired predisposition for developing some of the most common forms of cancer may be at a considerably greater risk than need be because of their fat intake. If this proves to be the case (and proving this is where a major problem lies), it would be a serious situation, indeed. Epidemiological surveys have provided support for linking higher rates of several common forms of cancer to higher fat intakes (Wynder, Bross, Hirayama 1960; Carroll, Plunkett, Gammal 1968). Animal experiments show that the incidence of certain types of tumors can be substantially lowered by manipulating dietary fat, particularly unsaturated fat (Chan, Cohen 1974). The reports by Drs. Bandura Reddy, Daniel Longnecker, Bill Roebuck, Homer Black and Margaret King will emphasize the extent to which the occurrence of tumors in animal organs, which are also frequent sites of neoplasia in humans, can be modified by adjusting the amount of fat consumed. These effects of modifying dietary fat have been shown not to be due to caloric density changes or to fiber content. Rather the effects appear to be due to fat itself, especially unsaturated fat. A number of unanswered questions remain. For example, does the dietary fat-enhanced incidence of various types of tumors occur through the same mechanism? Is the critical time during which dietary fat influences tumor development the same for various tumor types? Are certain types of tumors affected only by unsaturated fat and not by saturated fat or total fat, and would that difference signify that the mechanisms involved in the enhancement are not the same? Is the effect of elevated dietary fat on carcinogenesis the result of an imbalance between unsaturated fat and other dietary components such as antioxidants or micronutrients like selenium? How low would a low fat diet have to be for the enhancement of tumorigenesis to be minimized in humans if the incidence is, indeed, augmented by dietary fat? Can the fat consumed in a diet that averages out as low-fat be relatively high part of the time and very low part of the time and still have the same benefit of a diet that has a constantly low fat content? Will a low fat diet be beneficial to individuals who have developed metastatic disease? Is the influence of dietary fat only on the rate of growth of tumors rather than on the initiation process, or both, and does this apply to all types of tumors affected by dietary fat? Is the effect of fat in the target organ itself or is it exerted through other systems, such as the endocrines or the mixed oxidase function systems of the immune system?

Some of these questions will be addressed in this session, and insights provided should be helpful in designing new experiments to acquire more definitive information to focus the mechanism or mechanisms through which dietary fat influences tumorigenesis. It may not be necessary to understand the mechanism to determine how to apply the information which has been gained to reduce the risk of cancer in human beings, but an understanding of mechanism may be necessary to determine when and how dietary intervention may be required. An understanding of mechanism could result in an entirely different, perhaps more practical approach than a complete change in dietary habits for the purpose of cancer prevention.

The research in the area of nutrition and cancer has developed into a body of information that now enables rational approaches to mechanism to be made, at least in animal models, For example, in one tumor model, the full effect of dietary fat is expressed when only 3% linoleic acid (as total fat) is present in the diet (Hopkins, Kennedy, Carroll 1980). Higher levels of unsaturated fat did not increase tumor incidence. This suggests that prostaglandins could be involved in the enhancement effect and data exists supporting this (Honn, Bockman, Marnett 1981). But the effect of linoleic acid in this model could be species specific or limited to a single type of carcinogen. Indeed, most human dietary intake includes more than 3% linoleic acid, yet incidences of specific types of tumor vary widely, world-wide, and correlate more significantly with total fat intake. If several mechanisms are involved in the increased tumorigenesis caused by dietary fat, it is possible that in some types of cancer, modification of the type of fat consumed rather than of the total intake of fat could have prevention value.

There are a number of ways in which dietary fat might alter the carcinogenic process and the problem is not so much one of constructing hypotheses as one of determining which hypothesis is most likely to reveal new insights if examined by laboratory investigation. Fat consumption may influence the absorption and distribution of a carcinogen; sites of deposition and metabolism could be influenced by the fatty acid composition of cell membranes which is readily modified by the type of fatty acids present in the dietary fat consumed. This, in turn, could modify the dynamic balances of function required for healthy tissues. It is unlikely, however, that the influence of dietary fat on tumorigenesis will be an effect solely of fat alone.

It seems more likely that nutrient interactions of various food constituents will also be involved. The primary obstacle to an understanding of the effect of dietary fat and other dietary components on cancer development continues to revolve around our incomplete understanding of the carcinogenic process. Until such an understanding is achieved, specific answers to the question of the role of diet in modifying the carcinogenic process are likely to be slow in coming. Nevertheless, it is entirely possible that a better understanding of the carcinogenic process itself will develop from the nutritional approach.

REFERENCES

Aries V, Crowther JS, Drasar BS, Hill MJ, Williams REO (1969). Bacteria and the aetiology of cancer of the large bowel. Gut 10:334.

Artman NR (1969). The chemical and biological properties of heated and oxidized fats. In Paoletti R, Kritchevsky D (eds): "Advances in Lipid Research," New York: Academic Press, p. 245.

Atlas SA, Boobis AR, Felton JB, Thorgeirsson SS, Nebert DW (1977). Ontogenetic expression of polycyclic aromatic compound-inducible monoxygenase activities and forms of cytochrome P-450 in rabbit. Evidence for temporal control and organ specificity of two genetic regulatory systems. J Biol Chem 252:4712.

Bast RC, Whitlock JP, Miller H, Rapp HJ, Gelboin HV (1974). Aryl hydrocarbon (benzo(a)pyrene) hydroxylase in human peripheral blood monocytes. Nature 250:664.

Becking GC (1976). Hepatic drug metabolism in iron-, magnesium-, and potassium-deficient rats. Fed Proc 35: 2480.

Campbell TC, Hayes JR (1976). The effect of quantity and quality of dietary protein on drug metabolism. Fed Proc 35:2470.

Carroll KK, Khor HT (1970). Effects of dietary fat and dose level of 7,12-dimethylbenz(α)anthracene on mammary tumor incidence in rats. Cancer Res 30:2260.

Carroll KK, Khor HT (1971). Effects of level and type of dietary fat on incidence of mammary tumors induced in female Sprague-Dawley rats by 7,12-dimethylbenz(α)-anthracene. Lipids 6:415.

Carroll KK, Plunkett ER, Gammal EB (1968). Dietary fat and mammary cancer. Can Med Assoc J 98:590.

Chan P-C, Cohen LA (1974). Effect of dietary fat, anti-estrogen, and antiprolactin on the development of mammary tumors in rats. J Natl Cncer Inst 52:25.

Dunning WF, Curtis MR, Maun ME (1949). The effect of dietary fat and carbohydrate on diethylstilbestrol-induced mammary cancer in rats. Cancer Res 9:354.

Gammal EB, Carroll KK, Plunkett ER (1967). Effects of dietary fat on the uptake and clearance of 7,12-dimethylbenz(α)anthracene by rat mammary tissue. Cancer Res 27:1737.

Guengerich FP (1977). Separation and purification of multiple forms of microsomal cytochrome P-450. Activities of different forms of cytochrome P-450 towards several components of environmental interest. J Biol Chem 252: 3970.

Hietanen E, Laitinen M, Vanio H, Hanninen O (1974). Dietary fats and properties of endoplasmic reticulum: II. Dietary lipid induced changes in actitivies of drug metabolizing enzymes in liver and duodenum of rat. Lipids 10:467.

Honn KV, Bockman RS, Marnett LJ (1981). Prostaglandins and cancer: A review of tumor initiation through tumor metastasis. Prostaglandins 21:833.

Hopkins GJ, Kennedy JG, Carroll KK (1980). Polyunsaturated fatty acids as promoters of mammary carcinogenesis induced in Sprague-Dawley rats by 7,12-dimethylbenz(α)anthracene. J Natl Cancer Inst 66:517.

Huang M-T, West SB, Lu AYH (1976). Separation, purification, and properties of multiple forms of cytochrome P-450 from the liver microsomes of phenobarbital-treated mice. J Biol Chem 251:4659.

Levin W, Conney AH, Alvares AP (1972). Induction of benzo[α]pyrene hydroxylase in human skin. Science 176:419.

Miller EC, Miller JA, Hartmann H (1961). N-hydroxy-2-acetylaminofluorene: A metabolite of 2-acetylaminofluorene with increased carcinogenic activity in the rat. Cancer Res 21:815.

Miller JA (1970). Carcinogenesis by Chemicals - An Overview. Cancer Res 30:559.

Miller JA, Miller EC (1969). The metabolic activation of carcinogenic aromatic amines and amides. Progr in Tumor Res 11:273.

Nebert DW, Gelboin HV (1969). The in vivo and in vitro induction of aryl hydrocarbon hydroxylase in mammalian cells of different species, tissues, strains and development and hormonal states. Arch Biochem. Biophys 134:76.

Nebert DW, Winker J, Gelboin HV (1969). Aryl hydrocarbon hydroxylase activity in human placenta from cigarette smoking and nonsmoking women. Cancer Res 29:1763.

Newberne PM, Rogers AE (1973). Rat colon carcinomas associated with aflatoxin and marginal vitamin A. J Natl Cancer Inst 50:439.

Nigro ND, Singh DV, Campbell RL, Pak MS (1975). Effect of dietary beef fat on intestinal tumor formation by azoxymethane in rats. J Natl Cancer Inst 54:439.

Norred WP, Wade AE (1972). Dietary fatty acid-induced alterations of hepatic microsomal drug metabolism. Biochem Pharmacol 21:2287.

Omura T, Sato R, Cooper DY, Rosenthal O, Estabrook RW (1965). Function of cytochrome P-450 of microsomes. Fed Proc 24:1181.

Reddy BS, Weisberger JH, Wynder EL (1974). Effects of dietary fat level and dimethylhydrazine on fecal acid and neutral sterol excretion and colon carcinogenesis in rats. J Natl Cancer Inst 52:507.

Rodgers AE, Newberne PM (1973). Dietary enhancement of intestinal carcinogenesis by dimethylhydrazine in rats. Nature 246:491.

Roffo AH (1946). Carcinogenic value of oxidated oils. Amer J Digest Dis 13:33.

Sugai M, Witting LA, Tsuchujama H, Kummerow FA (1962). The effect of heated fat on the carcinogenic activity of 2-acetylaminofluorene. Cancer Res 22:510.

Tannenbaum A (1942). The Genesis and Growth of Tumors. III. Effects of high fat diets. Cancer Res 2:468.

Watson AF, Mellanby E (1980). Tar cancer in mice. II. The condition of the skin when modified by external treatment or diet, as a factor in influencing the cancerous reaction. Brit J Exp Path 11:209.

Whitlock JP, Cooper HL, Gelboin HV (1972). Aryl hydrocarbon (benzopyrene) hydroxylase is stimulated in human lymphocytes by mitogens and benz(α)anthracene. Science 177:618.

Wynder EL, Bross LJ, Hirayama T (1960). A study of the epidemiology of cancer of the breast. Cancer 13:559.

Zannoni VG, Sato, PH (1976). The effect of certain vitamin deficiencies on hepatic drug metabolism. Fed Proc 35: 2464.

Diet, Nutrition, and Cancer:
From Basic Research to Policy Implications, pages 17–31
© *1983 Alan R. Liss, Inc., 150 Fifth Avenue, New York, NY 10011*

DIETARY LIPIDS AND THEIR RELATIONSHIP TO COLON CANCER

Bandaru S. Reddy

American Health Foundation
Naylor Dana Institute for Disease Prevention
Valhalla, New York   10595

During the past two decades, epidemiologic studies have investigated the influence of environmental factors on the occurance of colon cancer. Reliable data obtained from select and scientifically sound cancer registries suggest that diets particularly high in total fat and low in certain fibers, vegetables, and micronutrients are generally associated with an increased incidence of colon cancer (Armstrong and Doll 1975, Burkitt 1978, Correa and Haenszel 1978, Graham and Mettlin 1979). Dietary fat may be a risk factor in the absence of factors that are protective, such as use of high fibrous foods and fiber (Graham and Mettlin 1979, Reddy et al. 1980a, Reddy et al. 1978).

This brief review evaluates not only current experimental research on the relation between the dietary lipids and colon cancer, but also various initiators and promoters involved in colon carcinogenesis. Finally, it presents an evaluation of the mechanism whereby dietary lipids modulate to high risk for the development of this important cancer.

ETIOLOGY OF COLON CANCER

Cancer of the colon has been the subject of several epidemiologic reviews (Correa and Haenszel 1978). The major differences in intra-country and inter-country distribution and in migrants, as well as differences in religious groups of this cancer suggest that the nutritional factors and lifestyles are important in the incidence and mortality (Correa and Haenszel 1978, MacMahon et al. 1980, Haenszel et al. 1973).

The possible relationship between dietary factors and colon cancer, has been investigated by correlational, case-control and cohort studies. Wynder and Reddy (1973) proposed that colon cancer incidence is mainly associated with total dietary fat. A worldwide correlation between colon cancer incidence and total fat consumption has been established (Carroll and Khor 1975). Enig et al. (1978) examined the fat-cancer relationship in the United States and found an equally strong, significant positive correlation of colon cancer with total fat and vegetable fat. Several investigators have shown that the dietary variables chiefly associated with large bowel cancer rates were meat and total fat (Armstrong and Doll 1975). In general, these results support a role for total dietary fat in the incidence of colon cancer.

Studies attempting to explain the frequency of large bowel cancer have used both correlation and case-control studies. Wynder et al. (1969) conducted a large-scale retrospective study on large-bowel cancer patients in Japan, which suggested a correlation between the Westernization of the Japanese diet and colon cancer. Haenszel et al. (1973) demonstrated an association between colon cancer and dietary beef in Hawaiian Japanese cases and controls. A case-control study of cancer of the colon in Canada indicated an elevated risk for those with an increased intake of calories, total fat and saturated fat (Jain et al. 1980).

The studies cited led us to accept diet as a major etiologic factor in colon cancer. Diets high in total fat, and low in fiber are associated with an increased incidence of colon cancer in man. High dietary fiber acts as a protective factor in population consuming a high amount of total fat.

CONCEPT OF DIETARY FAT AND COLON CANCER

Aries et al. (1969) have suggested that (a) the amount of dietary fat determines the levels of intestinal bile acids as well as the composition of the gut microflora, and (b) the gut microflora metabolize these acid sterols to tumorigenic compounds active in the colon. Reddy et al. (1980a) suggested that the dietary fat increases the excretion of bile acids into the gut, as well as modifies the activity of gut microflora which enhances the formation of secondary bile acids in the colon. These secondary bile acids act as tumor promoters in the colon (Reddy et al. 1980a).

Studies were carried out in our laboratory and elsewhere on the excretion of bile acids in high- and low-risk population for colon cancer development. This subject has been reviewed recently (Reddy 1981a, Reddy 1981b). Briefly, the population with a high risk for colon cancer has an increased amount of colonic secondary bile acids, namely deoxycholic acid and lithocholic acid. In addition, people on a high-fat diet appear to have a higher level of fecal secondary bile acids compared to those on a low-fat diet.

Until recently, there were no concepts on the nature of the genotoxic carcinogens associated with the etiology of colon cancer. Based on the discovery of Sugimura et al. (1982) that there were powerful mutagens on the surface of fried meat, Weisburger et al. (1980) proposed that these mutagens may be carcinogens responsible for colon cancer. Weisburger et al. (1980) also demonstrated that the fat content of food may also play a role in the mutagen formation. Several of these fried meat mutagens are similar to the aromatic amines related to 3,2'-dimethyl-4-aminobiphenyl (DMAB) which is experimental colon carcinogen in animal models. Experiments on the effects of feeding mice on diets containing fried meat mutagens such as Trp-p-1 or Trp-p-2 demonstrated the hepatocarcinogenicity of these compounds (Sugimura 1982). However, the carcinogen activity of fried meat mutagens for the colon remains to be determined.

The search for mutagenic activity in the feces has been stimulated by the need to understand the nature of genotoxic compounds, if any, relevant to colon cancer. These studies demonstrate that the populations who are at high-risk for colon cancer and consuming either a high-fat and/or non-vegetarian diet excrete increased amount of fecal mutagens compared to low-risk population (Ehrich et al. 1979, Bruce et al. 1977, Kuhnlein et al. 1981, Reddy et al. 1980a, Mower (1982). Studies are in progress in many laboratories to isolate and identify these fecal mutagens and to determine their carcinogenic activity.

Based on the above information, it has been suggested that (a) the extent of the carcinogenic stress from the exogenous source is probably rather weak, (b) high fat diet alters concentration of bile acids and the activity of gut microflora which may in turn produce tumor-promoting substances from bile acids in the lumen of the colon, (c) certain dietary fibers not only enhance binding of tumorigenic compounds in the gut, but also dilute them so that their effect on the colonic mucosa is minimal, and (d) dietary fat, fiber and certain vegetables modify the intestinal mucosal as well as hepatic enzyme inhibitors or inducers that alter the capacity of the animal or man to metabolize the tumorigenic compounds (Reddy et al. 1980a, Hill et al. 1971, Goldin and Gorbach 1976, Campbell 1979; Table 1).

EXPERIMENTAL STUDIES IN ANIMAL MODELS

Studies on the mechanisms of colon carcinogenesis have been assisted by the discovery of several animal models in which chemically-induced colon tumors show the type of lesions observed in man. The animal models are now being used effectively to study the multiple environmental factors involved in the pathogenesis of colon cancer.

Dietary Fat and Colon Carcinogenesis

Nigro et al. (1975) induced intestinal tumors in male Sprague-Dawley rats by subcutaneous administration of azoxymethane (AOM) and compared animals fed Purina chow with 35% beef fat to those fed Purina chow containing 5% fat. Animals fed the high fat developed more intestinal tumors and more metastasis into abdominal cavity, lungs and liver than the rats fed the low-fat diet. In another study, W/Fu rats fed a 30% lard diet had an increased number of 1,2-dimethylhydrazine(DMH)-induced colon tumors compared to the animals fed the standard diet (Bansal et al. 1978). Rats fed a diet high in beef fat (28%, with enough corn oil (2%) to prevent essential fatty acid deficiency) or a diet marginally deficient in lipotropes but high in fat were significantly more susceptible to DMH-induced colon tumors than those fed a low-fat diet (Rogers and Newberne 1973, 1975). These

Table 1.   Modifying Factors in Colon Cancer

Dietary Fat[a]	Dietary Fibers[a,b]	Micronutrients (include vitamins minerals, antioxidants, etc.)
1. Increases bile acid secretion into gut	1. Certain fibers increase fecal bulk and dilute carcinogens and pro-motors	1. Modify carcinogenesis at activation and detoxification level
2. Increases metabolic activity of gut bacteria	2. Modify metabolic activity of gut bacteria	2. Act also at promotional phase of carcinogenesis
3. Increases secondary bile acids in colon that act as tumor promoters	3. Modify the metabolism of carcinogens and/or promoters	
4. Alters immune system		
5. Stimulation of mixed function oxidase system		

a   Dietary factors, particularly high total dietary fat and a relative lack of certain dietary fibers and vegetables have a role.

b   High dietary fiber or fibrous foods may be a protective factor even in the high dietary fat intake.

results suggest that total dietary fat may have a function in the pathogenesis of experimentally-induced colon cancer.

Reddy et al. (1976a) designed experiments to study the effect of a type and amount of dietary fat for two generations before animals were exposed to treatment with a carcinogen. Animals fed the diets containing 20% lard or 20% corn oil were more susceptible to colon tumor induction by DMH than those fed 5% lard or 5% corn oil (Table 2). The type of fat appears to be immaterial at the 20% level, although at the 5% fat level, the unsaturated fat (corn oil) predisposes to more DMH-induced colon tumors than saturated fat (lard). Broitman et al. (1977) showed that rats fed a 20% safflower oil diet had more DMH-induced large bowel tumors than the animals fed either the 5% or 20% coconut oil diets that are high in medium chain triglycerides. These studies suggest that dietary polyunsaturated fat per se is more effective than saturated fat high in medium chain triglycerides in augmenting tumorigenesis by DMH. However, these data indicate that at low dietary fat levels, diets rich in polyunsaturated fats are more effective tumor promoters than diets rich in saturated fats irrespective of the source of the saturated fat.

Investigations were also carried out to test the effect of high dietary fat on colon tumor induction by a variety of carcinogens, DMH, methylazoxymethanol (MAM) acetate, DMAB or methylnitrosurea (MNU), which not only differ in metabolic activation but also represent a broad spectrum of exogenous carcinogens (Reddy et al. 1977a, Reddy and Ohmori 1981). Irrespective of the colon carcinogen, animals fed a 20% fat diet had a greater incidence of colon tumors than did rats fed a diet containing 5% fat (Table 2).

The suggestion that promotion may be involved in intestinal cancer has been supported by the observation that the carcinogenic response to a variety of intestinal carcinogens is enhanced by the dietary fat which in itself is not carcinogenic. Recent studies indicate that the enhanced tumorigenesis in the animals fed the high-fat diet is due to promotional effects (Bull et al. 1979). Ingestion of high-fat diet increased the intestinal tumor incidence when fed after AOM administration,

Table 2. Colon Tumor Incidence in Rats Fed Diets High in Fat and Treated with Colon Carcinogens

% of dietary fat	% of protein as casein	Carcinogen	% of rats with colon tumors
Lard			
5	25	DMH[a]	17
20	25	DMH	67
Corn Oil			
5	25	DMH[a]	36
25	25	DMH	64
Beef Fat			
5	22	DMH[b]	27
20	22	DMH	60
5	22	MNU[c]	33
20	22	MNU	73
5	22	MAM acetate[d]	45
20	22	MAM acetate	80
5	20	DMAB[e]	26
20	20	DMAB	74

a Female F344 rats, at 7 weeks of age, were given DMH s.c. at a weekly dose rate of 10 mg per kg body weight for 20 weeks, and autopsied 10 weeks later.

b Male F344 rats, at 7 weeks of age, were given a single s.c. dose of DMH, 150 mg per kg body weight, and autopsied 30 weeks later.

c Male F344 rats, at 7 weeks of age, were given MNU i.r., 2.5 mg per rat, twice a week for 2 weeks and autopsied 30 weeks later.

d Male F344 rats, at 7 weeks of age, were given a single i.p. dose of MAM acetate, 35 mg per kg body weight, and autopsied 30 weeks later

e Male F344 rats, at 7 weeks of age, were given DMAB s.c. at a weekly dose rate of 50 mg per kg body weight for 20 weeks, and autopsied 20 weeks later.

but not during or before AOM treatment. Therefore, the high-fat diet in this model exhibited most of the properties of promoters. The carcinogenic process in the human may have similar characteristics. The fact that ubiquitous environmental carcinogens are present at very low concentrations suggests that promoting factors may have a preponderant influence on the eventual outcome of the neoplastic process in humans.

Bile Acids and Colon Tumor Promotion

More recently, cholecystectomy, a procedure that increases the concentration of secondary bile acids in feces, has been shown to predispose to the development of cancer of right-sided colon in humans (Linos et al. 1981). One of the changes associated with cholecystectomy is an increased proportion of secondary bile acids such as deoxycholic acid and lithocholic acid in the total bile acid pool, this change being due to the increased enterohepatic recycling and the exposure of bile acids to gut bacteria.

The role of bile acids in colon tumor promotion has received support from studies in animal models. Chomchai et al. (1974) demonstrated that the carcinogenic effect of AOM in rats was increased by surgically diverting bile to the middle of the small intestine, a procedure that also raised the fecal excretion of bile salts. The evidence of the importance of bile acids as colon tumor promoters came from our studies (Narisawa et al. 1974, Reddy et al. 1976b Reddy et al. 1977b, 1977c, Reddy and Watanabe 1979). The development of colon tumors increased significantly among those conventional rats initiated with limited amounts of intrarectal MNNG to give a definite low yield of colon cancer and administered with intrarectal, deoxycholic acid, lithocholic acid or taurodeoxycholic acid as promoters, compared with the group that was given only the carcinogen. The bile acids themselves did not produce any tumors. A recent study also indicates that the primary bile acids, cholic acid and chenodeoxycholic acid given intrarectally to conventional rats also increased MNNG-induced colon tumors and these primary bile acids are converted to deoxycholic acid and lithocholic acid, respectively. Cohen et al. (1980) reported that cholic acid in the diet increased MNU-induced colon carcinogenesis in rats. Total fecal bile acids, particuarly deoxycholic acid output, were elevated in animals fed cholic acid as compared with controls. This increase in fecal deoxycholic acid was due to bacterial 7α-dehydroxylation of cholic acid in the colonic contents. These studies demonstrate that these secondary bile acids have a promoting effect in colon carcinogenesis.

The mechanism of action of bile acids in colon carcinogenesis has not been elucidated. Bile acids have been shown to affect cell kinetics in the intestinal epithelium (Bagheri et al. 1978). The cell renewal system is dynamic and may be influenced by changes in a number of factors, including bile acids in the intestine. Recently, Cohen et al. (1980) reported an enhanced colonic cell proliferation in rats fed cholic acid, as well as in animals treated with intrarectal MNU. Lipkin (1975) demonstrated that, during neoplastic transformation of colonic cells, a similar sequence of changes leading to uncontrolled proliferative activity develops in colon cancer in humans and in rodents given a colon carcinogen. Recent studies of Takano et al. (1981) suggest that the induction of colonic epithelial ornithine decarboxylase and S-adenosyl-L-methionine decarboxylase activities by the bile acids may play a role in these mechanisms. This study indicates that the colonic epithelial responses of the polyamine biosynthetic enzymes, to applications of bile acids are among the earliest changes to occur in this tissue in response to promoting agents.

Sterols and Colon Carcinogenesis

Recent studies have indicated that lowering of serum cholesterol levels is associated with increased colon cancer risk in humans (Williams et al. 1981). Whether low serum cholesterol levels in these patients precede or follow colon cancer is not completely determined. It is possible that this relationship might not be to low serum cholesterol, but due to delivery of bile salts to the intestinal tract resulting from the techniques used to lower serum cholesterol.

Cruse et al. (1979) proposed that prolonged exposure of dietary cholesterol is cocarcinogenic for human colon cancer, in that it facilitates the development, growth, and spread of the disease because dietary fats promote the action of several experimental carcinogens. Broitman et al. (1977) demonstrated that the interaction between dietary polyunsaturated fat and dietary cholesterol and or tissue cholesterol may promote tumorigenesis when compared with dietary saturated fat and cholesterol in the animal model.

Cholesterol $3\beta,5\alpha,6\beta$-triol (triol), a principal metabolite of cholesterol epoxide, has been found in increased levels in feces of patients of colon cancer and ulcerative colitis (Reddy et al. 1977b, Reddy and Wynder 1977). Bischoff (1969) has reviewed the carcinogenic effects of steroids and reported that cholesterol epoxide was carcinogenic in both rats and mice, but not carcinogenic to the colon. Cholesterol, cholesterol epoxide, and triol were not found to exert any colon tumor-promoting activity in both germfree and conventional rat models (Reddy and Watanabe 1979). These observations suggest that cholesterol or its metabolites produced by the colonic bacteria are not detectably either a carcinogen or a promoter to the colonic mucosa.

The possible role of β-sitosterol, a plant sterol, in colon tumor development has been studied by Cohen et al (1982). Rats given MNU and fed β-sitosterol at 0.2% level had significantly fewer colon tumors compared to those given only MNU. When β-sitosterol was added to the diet containing cholic acid, the tumor-promoting effect of cholic acid was inhibited in the animal model.

FUTURE STUDIES

1.   The dose-response relationship of fat (unsaturated and saturated) and its effect on the colon tumor incidence and latency period in animal models have not been studied. Many of the studies thus far have used a very high carcinogen dose which does not mimic the human situation where the carcinogenic stresss from the exogenous source is rather weak, and were unable to determine the difference between high- and low-fat in terms of latency period. Studies are warranted using low dose level of carcinogen and different levels of dietary fat to determine the dose-response effect of fat on the colon tumor incidence and latency period.

2. Recent epidemiologic studies suggest that decreased serum cholesterol may be associated with increased mortality of colon cancer. However, the evidence is equivocal. Well-controlled studies are warranted to investigate in both humans and in realistic animal models, the relationship between dietary cholesterol, serum cholesterol and colon cancer.

CONCLUSIONS

During the last decade, some progress has been made in the understanding of the role played by the dietary constituents in general and specifically the role of lipids in colon cancer. The epidemiologic studies on the relationship of lipids to colon cancer have been strengthened by the animal model studies. The populations with high incidence of cancer of the colon are characterized by consumption of a high level of dietary fat. Furthermore, dietary fat may be a risk factor for colon cancer in the absence of factors that are protective, such as use of high fibrous foods and cereals and whole grains. Thus, alteration of dietary habits leading to a lower intake of fat and higher intake of certain fibers would be indicated to decrease the risk of this important cancer.

Most human cancers in reality result from a complex interaction of carcinogens, co-carcinogens, and tumor promoters. However, the understanding of post-initiating events appears to offer some promise. Most of nutritional or dietary factors act at the promotional phase of carcinogenesis. Because promotion is a reversable process, in contrast to the rapid, irreversible process of initiation by carcinogens, manipulation of promotion would seem to be the best method of colon cancer prevention.

ACKNOWLEDGMENTS

This research was supported in part from grants CA-16382, CA-29602 and CA-17613, and contracts CP-85659 and CP-05605 from the National Cancer Institute. The author acknowledges the expert assistance of Ms. Arlene Banow in preparation of the manuscript.

REFERENCES

Aries V, Crowther JS, Drasar BS, Hill MJ, Williams REO
(1969). Bacteria and etiology of cancer of the large
bowel. Gut 10:334.

Armstrong D, Doll R (1975). Environmental factors and
cancer incidence and mortality in different countries
with special reference to dietary practices. Int J
Cancer 15:617.

Bagheri SA, Bolt MG, Boyer JL Palmer RH (1978).
Stimulation of thymidine incorporation in mouse liver
and biliary tract epithelium by lithocholate and deoxy-
cholate. Gastroenterol 7:188.

Bansal BR, Rhoads JE, Jr, Bansal SC (1978). Effects of
diet on colon carcinogenesis and the immune system in
rats treated with 1,2-dimethylhydrazine. Cancer Res
38:3293.

Bischoff F (1969). Carcinogenic effect of steroids.
Adv Lipid Res 7:165.

Bruce WR, Varghese AJ, Furrer R, Land PC (1977). A
mutagen in the feces of normal humans. In Hiatt HH,
Watson JP, Winston JA (eds): "Origins of Human
Cancer", Cold Spring Harbor Conf, Cell Proliferation 4,
1651.

Broitman SA, Vitale JJ, Vavrousek-Jakuba E, Gottlieb LS
(1977). Polyunsaturated fat, cholesterol and large
bowel tumorigenesis. Cancer 40:2455.

Bull AW, Soullier BK, Wilson PS, Hayden MT, Nigro ND
(1979). Promotion of azoxymethane-induced intestinal
cancer by high-fat diets in rats. Cancer Res 39:4956.

Burkitt DP (1978). Colonic-rectal cancer: fiber and
other dietary factors. Am J Clin Nutr 31:S58.

Campbell TC (1979). Influence of nutrition on metabolism
of carcinogenesis. Adv Nutr Res 2:29.

Carroll KK. Khor HT. (1975). Dietary fat in relation to
tumorigenesis. Prog Biochem Pharmacol 10:308.

Chomchai C, Bhadrachari.N, Nigro ND (1974). A rat model
for studying colonic cancer: Effect of cholestyramine
on induced tumors. Dis Colon Rectum 17:310.

Cohen BI, Raicht RF, Deschner EE, Takahashi M, Sarwal AN
Fazzini E (1980). Effect of cholic acid feeding on
N-methyl-N-nitrosourea-induced colon tumors and cell
kinetics in rats. J Natl Cancer Inst 64:573.

Cohen BI, Raicht RF, Islam A (1982). Effects of sterols
    and bile acids on colon tumor formation in rats. 1981
    Workshop on Large Bowel Cancer, Dallas, TX, 19.
Correa P, Haenszel W (1978). The epidemiology of large
    bowel cancer. Adv Cancer Res 26:1.
Cruse JP, Lewin MR, Clark CG (1979). Dietary cholesterol
    is co-carcinogenic for human colon cancer. Lancet
    1:152
Ehrich M, Ashell JE, Van Tassell RL, Wilkins TD,
    Walker, ARP, Richardson NJ (1979). Mutagens in the
    feces of 3 South African populations at different
    levels of risk for colon cancer. Mutat Res 64:231.
Enig MG, Mann RJ, Keeney M (1978). Dietary fat and
    cancer trends - a critique. Fed Proc 37:2215.
Goldin BR, Gorbach SL (1976). The relationship between
    diet and rat fecal bacterial enzymes implicated in
    colon cancer. J Natl Cancer Inst 57:371.
Graham S, Mettlin C (1979). Diet and colon cancer.
    Am J Epidemiol 109:1
Haenszel W, Berg JW, Segi M, Kurihara M, Locke FB (1973).
    Large bowel cancer in Hawaiian Japanese. J Natl Cancer
    Inst 51:1765.
Hill MJ, Drasar BS, Aries VC, Crowther JS, Hawksworth GB,
    Williams REQ (1971). Bacteria and etiology of cancer
    of large bowel. Lancet 1:95.
Jain M, Cook GM, Davis FG, Grace MG, Howe GR, Miller AB
    (1980). A case-control study of diet and colorectal
    cancer. Intl J Cancer 26:757.
Kuhnlein U, Bergstrom D, Kuhnlein H (1981). Mutations
    in feces from vegetarians and non-vegetarians. Mut Res
    85:1.
Linos DA, Beard CM, O'Fallon WM, Dockerty MB,
    Beart Jr. RW, Kurland LT (1981). Cholescystectomy and
    carcinoma of the colon. Lancet ii:379.
Lipkin M (1975). Present status and research frontiers.
    Cancer 36:2319.
MacMahon B, Copley G, Fraumeni Jr. JF, Greenwald P.
    Haenszel W (eds) (1980). "Populations at low risks of
    cancer" NCI monograph.
Mower HF, Ichinotsubo D, Wang LW, Mandel M, Stemmerman C
    Nomura A, Heilburn L (1982). Fecal mutagens in two
    Japanese populations with different colon cancer risks.
    Cancer Res 42:1164.

Narisawa T, Magadia NE, Weisburger JH, Wynder EL (1974).
Promoting effect of deoxycholic acid on colonic adenocarcinomas in germfree rats. J Natl Cancer Inst
53:1093.

Nigro ND, Singh DV, Campbell RL, Pak MS (1975). Effect
of dietary beef fat on intestinal tumor formation by
azoxymethane in rats. J Natl Cancer Inst 54:429.

Reddy BS (1981a). Dietary fat and its relationship to
large bowel cancer. Cancer Res 41:3700.

Reddy BS (1981b). Diet and excretion of bile acids.
Cancer Res 41:3766.

Reddy BS, Cohen L, McCoy GD, Hill P, Weisburger JH,
Wynder EL (1980a). Nutrition and its relationship to
cancer. In Klein G, Weinhouse S (eds): "Advances in
Cancer Research", 32, New York: Academic Press, p.
237.

Reddy BS, Hedges AR, Laakso K, Wynder EL (1978). Metabolic epidemiology of large bowel cancer. Fecal bulk
and constituents of high-risk North American and low-
risk Finnish populaton. Cancer 42:2832.

Reddy BS, Mangat S, Weisburger JH, Wynder EL (1977a).
Effect of high-risk diets for colon carcinogenesis or
intestinal mucosal and bacterial β-glucuronidase activity in F344 rats. Cancer Res 37:"3533.

Reddy BS, Martin CW, Wynder EL (1977b) Fecal bile acids
and cholesterol metabolites of patients with ulcerative
colitis, a high-risk group for colon cancer development. Can Res 37:1697.

Reddy BS, Narisawa T, Vukusich D, Weisburger, JH,
Wynder EL (1976a). Effect of quality and quantity of
dietary fat and dimethylhydrazine in colon carcinogenesis in rats. Proc Soc Exp Biol Med 151:237.

Reddy BS, Narisawa T, Weisburger JH, Wynder EL (1976b)
Promoting effect of deoxycholic acid on colonic adenocarcinomas in germfree rats. J Natl Cancer Inst
56:441.

Reddy BS, Ohmori T (1981). Effect of intestinal microflora and dietary fat on 3,2-dimethyl-4-aminobiphenly-
induced colon carcinogenesis in F344 rats. Cancer Res
41:1363.

Reddy BS, Sharma C, Darby L, Laakso K, Wynder EL (1980b).
Metabolic epidemiology of large bowel cancer: Fecal
mutagens in high- and low-risk population for colon
cancer, a preliminary report. Mut Res 72:511.

Reddy BS, Watanabe K (1979). Effect of cholesterol metabolites and promoting effect of lithocholic acid in
colon carcinogenesis in germfree and conventional F344
rats. Cancer Res 39:1521.

Reddy BS, Watanabe K, Weisburger JH, Wynder EL (1977c).
Promoting effect of bile acids in colon carcinogenesis
in germfree and conventional F344 rats. Cancer Res
37:3238.

Reddy BS, Wynder EL (1977). Metabolic epidemiology of
colon cancer: Fecal bile acids and neutral sterols in
colon cancer patients with adenomatous polyps. Cancer
39:2533.

Rogers AE, Newberne PM (1973). Dietary enhancement of
intestinal carcinogenesis by dimethylhydrazine in rats.
Nature (London) 246:491.

Rogers AE, Newberne PM (1975). Dietary effects on
chemical carcinogenesis in animal models for colon and
liver tumors. Cancer Res 35:3427.

Sugimura T (1982). Mutagens, carcinogens and tumor pro-
motors in in our daily food. Cancer 49:1970.

Takano S, Matsushima M, Erturk E, Bryan GT (1981).
Early induction of rat colonic epithelial ornithine and
S-adenyl-L-methionine decarboxylase activities by
N-methyl-N'-nitrosoguanidine or bile salts. Cancer Res
41:624.

Weisburger JH, Reddy BS, Spingarn NE, Wynder EL (1980).
Current views on the mechanisms involved in the eti-
ology of colorectal cancer. In Winawer S, Schottenfeld
D, Sherlock P. (eds). "Colorectal Cancer: Prevention,
Epidemiology and Screening", New York: Raven Press,
p 19.

Williams RR, Sorlie PD, Feinleib M, McNamara PM,
Kannel WB, Dawber TR (1981). Cancer incidence by
levels of cholesterol. JAMA 245:247.

Wynder EL, Kajitani T, Ishikawa S, Dodo H, Takano A.
(1969). Environmentalfactors of cancer of the colon
and rectum. II. Japanese epidemiological data. Cancer
23:1219.

Wynder EL, Reddy BS (1973). Studies of large bowel
cancer: human leads to experimental application. J
Natl Cancer Inst 50:1099.

Diet, Nutrition, and Cancer:
From Basic Research to Policy Implications, pages 33–47
© *1983 Alan R. Liss, Inc., 150 Fifth Avenue, New York, NY 10011*

DIETARY LIPID PROMOTION OF AZASERINE-INDUCED PANCREATIC
TUMORS IN THE RAT

B. D. Roebuck, Ph.D.

Assistant Professor of Toxicology
Department of Pharmacology and Toxicology

Daniel S. Longnecker, M.D.

Professor of Pathology
Department of Pathology
Dartmouth Medical School
Hanover, New Hampshire   03756

Epidemiologic studies have implicated several risk
factors which are associated with the development of
pancreatic carcinoma in humans. These include cigarette
smoking (Wynder 1975), exposure to specific chemicals
(Bates 1975), and dietary factors including fat content
(Wynder et al. 1973) and coffee consumption (MacMahon
et al. 1981). The specific components of cigarette smoke
which might cause pancreatic carcinoma have not been
identified although nitrosamines must be considered as
suspect because of experimental findings in animals.
Animal models for chemical induction of carcinomas in
rodents have been developed and studied in an attempt to
improve our understanding of carcinogenesis in the
pancreas (Reddy et al. 1979). More than a dozen
chemicals including several nitrosamines have been
identified which induce pancreatic carcinoma in several
rodent species. Two models have been more fully
characterized than the others. These are induction of
pancreatic carcinomas in Syrian golden hamsters by
N-nitrosobis(2-oxopropyl)amine (BOP) (Pour et al. 1981)
and in rats by azaserine (Longnecker et al. 1981).
Comparison of these models is of interest because Pour
regards the ductal or ductular cell as the origin of
carcinomas in BOP-treated hamsters, whereas we regard

acinar cells as the origin of carcinomas in the rat
model. Despite this proposed difference for histogenesis
of carcinomas, similar results have been obtained in
studies of the influence of dietary factors on
carcinogenesis in the two models. We have worked
primarily with the azaserine-rat model and it will be
described as background for the data presented below.

RAT-AZASERINE MODEL

Azaserine, O-diazoacetyl-L-serine, is a natural
antibiotic produced by a species of Streptomyces.
Azaserine is a mutagen in the Ames system (Staiano et al.
1980) and damages DNA at least in part by alkylation of
guanosine (Zurlo et al. 1982a). It is a direct acting
mutagen for bacteria, however, enzyme mediated steps
appear to be involved in its uptake and/or metabolism in
rodents. Recent work suggests that a pyridoxal dependent
enzyme system is involved (Zurlo et al. 1982b).

Azaserine has been given by intraperitoneal injection in most carcinogenesis experiments, however, it has
also induced pancreatic cancers after prolonged oral
administration. Earlier studies utilized regimens of 5
to 26 doses given over periods of 1 to 6 months, but we
have recently demonstrated that administration of a
single 30 mg/kg injection to 7 week old male Lewis rats
will induce carcinomas after a 15 to 18 month latent
period. The incidence of pancreatic carcinomas has
consistently been greater in male than in female rats by
a ratio of 2-3:1. Several rodent species and rat strains
have been compared in regard to sensitivity to induction
of pancreatic neoplasms by azaserine (Roebuck, Longnecker
1977). The Lewis strain of rats were more sensitive than
the Fisher 344 strain. Random bred Wistar rats are less
uniform in response to azaserine than Lewis rats although
most will respond. Other rat strains have not been
evaluated. Hamster, guinea pig and mouse are all less
responsive than rats to the induction of pancreatic
neoplasms by azaserine.

Beginning about two months following administration
of azaserine, multiple foci of phenotypically altered
acinar cells can be identified in the pancreas. In many
respects these lesions are comparable to early
carcinogen-induced foci in liver following administration

of hepatic carcinogens. These lesions, which have been
designated as atypical acinar cell nodules (AACN) have
been described and illustrated (Longnecker, Crawford
1974; Longnecker, Curphey 1975; Roebuck, Longnecker 1977).
Similar lesions have been described in the pancreas of
rats treated with several other pancreatic carcinogens.
Some AACN grow progressively achieving a diameter of 3 mm
by 4 months and 10 mm or more in studies of 12 months or
longer. Pancreatic weight is increased in azaserine-
treated rats in studies of 9 or more months duration.

Some of the rapidly growing lesions have compressed
the adjacent pancreas and are sometimes encapsulated.
These lesions have been designated as adenomas. There is
progressive dysplasia and anaplasia in other lesions so
that they appear to merit designation as "carcinoma-
in-situ". One year following initial azaserine treatment
we have encountered evidence of local invasion and/or
metastasis to liver, lung and skeletal muscle.

Most carcinomas maintain some evidence of acinar cell
differentiation although the lesions are pleomorphic and
often include duct-like, cystic and anaplastic areas. A
few tumors have been completely anaplastic, i.e. lacking
evidence of acinar or ductal differentiation. These
various histologic types have been described in detail
and illustrated (Longnecker et al. 1981).

Elsewhere in this volume the relationships of dietary
lipids to breast and colon carcinogenesis are discussed
in detail. The enhancement of carcinogenesis in these
two organs appears to be by promotion; however, experimental
carcinogenesis of the colon and breast is not nearly as
well characterized as the mouse skin system (Boutwell
1974). The analysis of the biochemical basis of promotion
in the mouse skin system is considerably advanced over all
other organ sites. The mouse skin was the first organ for
which promotion was demonstrated. The mouse skin system
enjoys at least two significant advantages over most other
target organs. First, the skin can continually be
monitored for appearance and progression of tumors.
Second, a pure chemical, 12-0-tetradecanoylphorbol-13-
acetate, is a known promoter of skin cancer and it has
been available in relatively pure form for many years (see
reviews, Boutwell 1974; Scribner, Suss 1978). In contrast,

we are not able to monitor continually the appearance and
progression of neoplasms in pancreas as can be done in
experimental skin and breast carcinogenesis. Serial
sacrifices which require much larger experimental groups
would be necessary for such experiments. We also lack a
specific chemical promoter for pancreatic carcinogenesis.

DIETARY MODULATION OF PANCREATIC CARCINOGENESIS

     In 1976, we began studies into the dietary modulation
of pancreatic cancer. Dietary lipids were but one of the
nutrients evaluated. As discussed above, there is a
dearth of etiologic clues to the cause of human pancreatic
adenocarcinoma. Epidemiologic data have suggested a
correlation between level of dietary fat consumption and
the incidence of pancreatic cancer (Wynder et al 1973;
Wynder 1975; Carroll, Khor 1975). However, dietary lipids
have not been the primary focus of any epidemiologic study
of pancreatic cancer.

Dietary Lipids

     Our initial experiments were designed to evaluate the
effects of various diets on azaserine-induced pancreatic
carcinogenesis in the rat (Roebuck et al. 1981a).
Separation of carcinogenesis into an initiation phase and
postinitiation phase was not attempted. Beginning at 4
weeks of age, male Lewis rats were injected i.p. with 10
mg azaserine/kg once per week for six successive weeks and
monthly thereafter until week 50. The total azaserine
dose was 160 mg/kg. From weaning, at 3 weeks of age, until
the termination of the experiment, all rats were fed a
powdered, purified test diet ad libitum. The control diet
(AIN) was the AIN-76 purified diet for rat and mouse which
was modified by the omission of the antioxidant ethoxyquin
(Report of the American Institute of Nutrition, 1977).
The test diets were modifications of the AIN diet. Table
1 gives the composition and caloric density of the diets.
One year following the first azaserine treatment, rats
were autopsied, the pancreases were weighed, fixed and
processed by standard histological techniques, and stained
with hematoxylin and eosin. The pancreases were examined
by light microscopy for adenomas and adenocarcinomas as
previously described (Longnecker et al. 1981). The
results of this study are summarized in Tables 2 and 3.

Table 1. Composition of Test Diets (% by weight)

Ingredient	AIN	Unsaturated fat	Saturated fat	Safflower oil
Casein	20.0	20.0	20.0	20.0
Methionine	0.3	0.3	0.3	0.3
Cornstarch	15.0	11.7	11.7	11.7
Sucrose	50.0	38.3	38.3	38.3
Cellulose	5.0	5.0	5.0	5.0
Corn oil	5.0	20.0	2.0	0.0
Coconut oil (hydrogenated)	0.0	0.0	18.0	0.0
Safflower oil	0.0	0.0	0.0	20.0
Vitamin mix[a]	1.0	1.0	1.0	1.0
Mineral mix[a]	3.5	3.5	3.5	3.5
Choline	0.2	0.2	0.2	0.2
Caloric content (kcal/g diet)	3.86	4.61	4.61	4.61

[a] The composition of the vitamin and mineral mixtures are those recommended by the Report of the American Institute of Nutrition (1977).

Treatment with azaserine (aza) or with saline is indicated in parentheses following the name of the diet. From Table 2, we conclude that rats fed the 20% fat diets, unsaturated fat and saturated fat, consumed more calories and attained a higher final body weight than the rats fed the 5% fat, AIN diet. In fact, the saturated fat (aza) group had a significantly greater caloric intake and attained a larger final body weight than the unsaturated fat(aza) group. The incidence and multiplicity of pancreatic adenomas and adenocarcinomas was significantly larger in the unsaturated fat(aza) group than the saturated fat(aza) or the AIN(aza) groups (Table 3). The difference between the unsaturated fat(aza) and AIN(aza) group could be due to differences in caloric intake and rate of growth; however, that clearly is not an explanation for the difference compared to the saturated fat(aza) group.

Table 2. Caloric Intake and Weights of Rats in the
Various Treatment Groups.

Caloric intake was calculated from the 24-hour food
consumption data and the caloric content of the various
diets. Food consumption was measured approximately every
other week starting at Week 6 and ending at Week 52 of the
experiment. The final body weights are based on the
numbers of rats listed in Table 3.

Treatment	Caloric Intake (kcal/24 hour)	Final body wt(g)
AIN(saline)...................	93 ± 11^a	670 ± 81^a
AIN(aza)......................	98 ± 13	$661 \pm 81_b$
Unsaturated fat(aza)..........	$106 \pm 11_{bc}$	846 ± 91^b
Saturated fat(aza)............	119 ± 19^{bc}	968 ± 112^{bc}

[a] Mean $\pm$ SD
[b] Greater than the AIN(aza) group ($p<0.05$).
[c] Greater than the unsaturated fat(aza) groups ($p<0.05$).

To further investigate the mechanisms of enhancement
by dietary unsaturated fat, we have divided the carcinogenesis experiments into two operational phases: initiation and postinitiation (Roebuck et al. 1981b). During the
initiation phase, male Lewis rats were injected with
azaserine (10 mg/kg) weekly for 6 to 8 weeks. The postinitiation phase began one week following the last azaserine dose. The diets fed and the azaserine dose during
the initiation phase and the diets fed and the duration of
the postinitiation phase are shown in Table 4. The
composition of the diets are those presented in Table 1.
If the saturated or unsaturated fat diet is fed during the
initiation phase and the AIN diet during the postinitiation phase, the incidence and mean number of pancreatic
tumors did not statistically differ from a similar group
fed the AIN diet during azaserine treatment. Dietary fat
had no effect on the initiation of pancreatic cancer by
azaserine.

Table 3. Dietary Modulation of Azaserine-induced
          Carcinogenesis of the Pancreas

Initially, there were 20 male Lewis rats per group.
Rats were killed at 1 year following the initial azaserine
treatment.

Treatment	Rats/ Group	Pancreas wt(g)	Adenomas and Carcinomas Incidence (%)	Neoplasms/ pancreas (mean)
AIN(saline).....16		1.4 ± 0.3^a	0 (0)	0
AIN(aza)........17		2.6 ± 1.4	12 (71)	2.4
Unsaturated fat(aza)......18		4.7 ± 2.5	18 $(100)^b$	>10
Saturated fat(aza)......20		2.6 ± 0.8	15 (75)	2.4

[a] Mean $\pm$ SD
[b] Greater than in the AIN(aza) group ($p<0.05$, χ^2 test).

The results of two sets of experiments designed
to evaluated the effects of dietary fats on the
postinitiation processes are also shown in Table 4.
Promotion by unsaturated fats is demonstrated in three
separate experimental groups. Unsaturated fat diet (20%
corn oil) fed during the postinitiation phase yielded a
significantly higher incidence of pancreatic tumors, than
was observed in similarly initiated rats fed either the
saturated fat diet or the AIN diet. The more highly
unsaturated diet of 20% safflower oil appeared to be more
effective as a promoting agent than the 20% corn oil diet
(Table 5).

Recently, Birt et al. (1981) have shown that Syrian
golden hamsters treated with a single dose of BOP and
subsequently fed diets of various corn oil levels have an
enhanced incidence and multiplicity of pancreatic ductular

Table 4. Effects of Dietary Fat on Initiation and Postinitiation Phases of Azaserine-induced Carcinogenesis in the Rat (From Roebuck et al. 1981b)

Initiation Phase		Postinitiation Phase			Pancreatic Adenomas and Adenocarcinomas	
Diet	Total Azaserine Dose at 10mg/kg	Diet	Duration (months)	Rats/group	Incidence (%)	Per pancreas (mean)
AIN	60	AIN	7.5	17	4 (24)	0.47
Saturated	60	AIN	7.5	18	2 (11)	0.11
Unsaturated	60	AIN	7.5	19	4 (21)	0.21
AIN	60	Saturated	7.5	20	3 (15)	0.20
AIN	60	Unsaturated	7.5	20	11 (55)[a]	1.45
AIN	80	AIN	10	18	10 (56)	0.9
AIN	80	Saturated	10	16	11 (69)	1.3
AIN	80	Unsaturated	10	17	16 (94)[b]	4.7
AIN	80	Safflower	10	17	16 (94)[b]	5.9[c]

[a] Compared to the AIN(aza)/AIN group (line 1), the AIN(aza)/unsaturated fat group (line 5) is significantly different (χ^2 test, $p < 0.05$).

[b] Compared to the AIN(aza)/AIN group (line 6), the AIN(aza)/unsaturated fat (line 8) and AIN(aza)/safflower oil (line 9) are significantly different (χ^2 test, $p < 0.05$).

[c] Two locally invasive pancreatic adenocarcinomas.

adenocarcinoma when fed 20.5% corn oil compared to lower levels of corn oil. Furthermore, the incidence of acinar cell nodules which are very rare in hamsters was elevated by the diets with higher corn oil content. Thus, the work of Birt et al. (1981) with another carcinogen and another species clearly complements our own observations.

Other Dietary Factors

The postinitiation phase of pancreatic carcinogenesis can be modulated by other dietary factors. A brief mention of these factors will serve to show that the pancreas is probably more similar to other organ systems than different. For example, we have observed that rats fed a chow diet had fewer and smaller azaserine-induced pancreatic lesions than a similar group of rats fed AIN diet (Longnecker et al. 1981). Experiments described in greater detail below indicated that this was a postinitiation effect. The inhibitory effects of chow type diets compared to purified diets have also been described in the 7,12-dimethylbenz(a)anthracene-induced rat breast tumor model (Chan, Dao 1981).

Retinoids are clearly chemopreventive agents by virtue of their effects during the postinitiation phase of a wide range of tumor models (Sporn, Newton 1979). In the rat-azaserine model, retinyl acetate (Longnecker et al. 1981), N-2-hydroxyethyl retinamide, N-4-propionyl-oxyphenyl retinamide, and retinylidene dimedone (Longnecker et al. 1982) have been shown to inhibit pancreatic carcinogenesis when fed during the postinitiation phase.

SHORT-TERM MODEL DEVELOPMENT

Quantitation of Preneoplastic Lesions

The incidence and number of pancreatic AACN have been used to predict the carcinogenic potential of azaserine in several rodent species and strains (Roebuck, Longnecker 1977). The pancreases of various azaserine-treated rodents were completely embedded by a standardized method so that AACN counted by light microscopy could be related to the true population of lesions in the entire pancreas. The AACN were then

expressed as number per pancreas. At 4 or 6 months
following the first azaserine injection and well before
cancers would be expected to arise, we were able to
correlate the number of AACN with the known sensitivity
of several species to azaserine-induced adenocarcinomas.
The predictive nature of AACN have been further
substantiated in additional rodent species (Roebuck,
Longnecker 1979) and under other conditions (Roebuck et
al. 1980). AACN counts versus various doses of azaserine
have yielded the dose-response curves shown in Figure 1
(Yager et al. 1981). The higher AACN counts at 6 versus
4 months probably reflect the detection of an increased
proportion of the nodule population because of growth of
nodules. Other studies (unpublished) indicate that a
single, 30 mg azaserine/kg injection at 14 days of age
will produce higher AACN counts than was observed in
either the 5 or 7 week old rats. At a known cytotoxic
dose (60 mg/kg) of azaserine, there was a decrease in the
number of AACN.

The measurement of the size of AACN in addition to
the number is valuable. In an experiment clearly showing
that azaserine-injected rats had more adenomas and
adenocarcinomas if concomitantly fed AIN diet versus
laboratory chow diet, the size of AACN (sq. mm, mean ±
SD) was larger in the AIN group (0.66 ± 0.19) than in the
chow group (0.20 ± 0.13). As discussed above, subsequent
count and size measurements of AACN showed that chow
inhibited carcinogenesis during the postinitiation phase
(Longnecker et al. 1981).

Effect of Dietary Lipids

The promotional effects of the unsaturated fat diet
is demonstrated by analysis of AACN number and size
(Table 5). At 4 months, but not at 2 months, following a
single dose of azaserine, more and larger AACN were
present in the rats fed unsaturated fat diet during the
postinitiation phase. These preliminary results further
demonstrate the utility of AACN as a predictor of
carcinogenicity. While these results are encouraging,
caution has to be expressed. First, occasionally a
nodule at least 10 times the area of all other nodules
will be detected. These are rare (1 per perhaps 20 rats)
and appear not to be related to the carcinogen treatment.

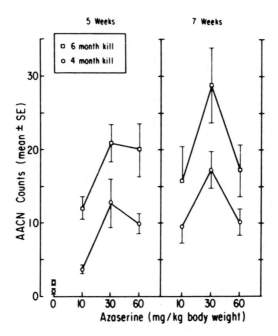

Figure 1. - Atypical acinar cell nodule (AACN) counts in rats as a function of age at injection, azaserine dose, and age at evaluation of AACN number. There were 10 rats per group and the bars represent the SD of the mean (From Yager et al. 1981).

Second, by our procedures, the probability of histologically sampling the larger AACN is greater and the probability of measuring the true size of any AACN is as yet unknown. This may be especially important in promotion studies where the treatment could increase either the number or size of nodules, or both. Campbell et al. (1982) have emphasized these aspects of morphometry with examples from hepatocarcinogenicity experiments.

CONCLUSIONS

High intakes of dietary unsaturated fats but not a saturated fat promotes pancreatic carcinogenesis.

Table 5. Effect of Dietary Unsaturated Fat on Counts and Size of Atypical Acinar Cell Nodules (AACN) Induced by Azaserine[a]

Postinitiation Phase	Atypical Acinar Cell Nodules (AACN)			
	2 months		4 months	
Dietary Treatments	Number	Size (sq.mm) x100	Number	Size (sq.mm) x100
AIN	5.4 ± 4.7[b]	1.86 ± 0.44	9.8 ± 8.1	4.02 ± 1.71
Saturated Fat	3.1 ± 2.7	1.71 ± 1.32	8.6 ± 6.7	5.44 ± 6.13
Unsaturated Fat	4.4 ± 3.7	1.83 ± 0.90	21.3 ± 7.4[c]	8.30 ± 3.68

a   Male, Lewis rats (10 per group) at 7 weeks of age were injected with a single dose of azaserine (10 mg/kg).

b   Mean ± SD

c $p < 0.05$ versus the AIN group

Unsaturated fat appears to enhance the growth of AACN. In short-term experiments of 4 months duration, AACN counts and size can be used as a predictive measure of either promotion or chemoprevention. Specific mechanisms of promotion of pancreatic carcinogenesis by dietary unsaturated fat remain unexplained.

ACKNOWLEDGEMENTS

We thank Dr. O. Ross McIntyre for reviewing this manuscript and Ms. Brenda Berube and the Norris Cotton Cancer Center, Dartmouth-Hitchcock Medical Center for assistance in preparation of the manuscript. Supported by USPHS-NCI Grants CA-19410 from the National Pancreatic Cancer Project and CA-26594 from the Diet, Nutrition and Cancer Program.

REFERENCES

Bates RR (1975). Chemical carcinogenesis and the pancreas. J Surg Oncol 7:143.

Birt DR, Salmasi S and Pour PM (1981). Enhancement of experimental pancreatic cancer in Syrian Golden hamsters by dietary fat. J Natl Cancer Inst 67:1327.

Boutwell RK (1974). The function and mechanism of promoters of carcinogenesis. CRC Critical Reviews in Toxicology 2:419.

Campbell MA, Pitot HC, Potter VR (1982). Application of quantitative stereology to the evaluation of enzyme-altered foci in rat liver. Cancer Res 42:465.

Carroll KK and Khor HT (1975). Dietary fat in relation to tumorigenesis. Progr Biochem Pharmacol 10:308.

Chan CP and Dao TL (1981). Enhancement of mammary carcinogenesis by a high-fat diet in Fischer, Long-Evans, and Sprague-Dawley rats. Cancer Res 41:164.

Longnecker DS and Crawford BG (1974). Hyperplastic Nodules and adenomas of exocrine pancreas in azaserine-treated rats. J Natl Cancer Inst 53:573.

Longnecker DS and Curphey TJ (1975). Adenocarcinoma of the pancreas in azaserine-treated rats. Cancer Res 35:2249.

Longnecker DS, Curphey TJ, Kuhlmann ET and Roebuck BD (1982). Inhibition of pancreatic carcinogenesis by retinoids in azaserine-treated rats. Cancer Res 42:19.

Longnecker DS, Roebuck BD, Yager JD Jr, Lilja HS and Siegmund B (1981). Pancreatic carcinoma in azaserine-treated rats: induction classification and dietary modulation of incidence. Cancer 47:1562.

MacMahon B, Yen S, Trichopoulos D, Warren K, Nardi G (1981). Coffee and cancer of the pancreas. N Engl J Med 304:630.

Pour PM, Runge RG, Birt D, Gingell R, Lawson T, Nagel D, Wallcave L and Salmasi SZ (1981). Current knowledge of pancreatic carcinogenesis in the hamster and its relevance to the human disease. Cancer 47:1573.

Reddy JK, Scarpelli DG, Rao MS (1979). Experimental pancreatic carcinogenesis. Thatcher N ed Advances in Medical Oncology, Research and Education, Digestive Cancer New York: Pergamon Press 9:99.

Report of the American Institute of Nutrition Ad Hoc Committee on Standards of Nutrional Studies. (1977) J Nutrition 107:1340.

Roebuck BD, Lilja HS, Curphey TJ and Longnecker DS (1980). Pathologic and biochemical effects of azaserine in inbred Wistar/Lewis rats and noninbred CD^r-1 mice. J Natl Cancer Inst 65:383.

Roebuck BD and Longnecker DS (1977). Species and rat strain variation in pancreatic nodule induction by azaserine. J Natl Cancer Inst 59:1273.

Roebuck BD and Longnecker DS (1979). Response of two rodents, Mastomys natalensia and Mystromys albicaudatus, to the pancreatic carcinogen azaserine. J Natl Cancer Inst 62:1269.

Roebuck BD, Yager JD and Longnecker DS (1981a). Dietary modulation of azaserine-induced pancreatic carcinogenesis in the rat. Cancer Res 41:888.

Roebuck BD, Yager JD, Longnecker DS and Wilpone SA (1981b). Promotion by unsaturated fat of azaserine -induced pancreatic carcinogenesis in the rat. Cancer Res 41:3961.

Scribner JD and Suss R (1978). Tumor initiation and promotion. Int Review Expt Pathol 18:137.

Sporn MB and Newton DL (1979). Chemoprevention of cancer with retinoids. Fed Proc 38:2528.

Staiano N, Everson RB, Cooney DA, Longnecker DS and Thorgeirsson SS (1980). Mutagenicity of D- and L-azaserine, 6-diazo-5-oxo-L-norleucine and N-(N-methyl-N-nitrosocarbamyl)-L-ornithine in the Salmonella test system. Mutation Res 79:387.

Wynder EL (1975). An epidemiological evaluation of the causes of cancer of the pancreas. Cancer Res 35:2228.

Wynder EL, Mabachi K, Maruchi N and Fortner JG (1973). Epidemiology of cancer of the pancreas. J Natl Cancer Inst 50:645.

Yager JD, Roebuck BD, Zurlo J, Longnecker DS, Weselcouch EO, Wilpone SA (1981). A single-dose protocol for azaserine initiation of pancreatic carcinogenesis in the rat. Int J Cancer 28:601.

Zurlo J, Curphey TJ, Hiley R and Longnecker DS (1982a). Identification of 7-carboxymethylguanine in DNA from pancreatic acinar cells exposed to azaserine. Cancer Res 42:1286.

Zurlo J, Roebuck BD, Rutkowski JV, Curphey TJ and Longnecker DS (1982b). Effect of pyridoxal deficiency on pancreatic DNA damage and nodule induction by azaserine. Proc Amer Assoc Cancer Res 23:68.

Diet, Nutrition, and Cancer:
From Basic Research to Policy Implications, pages 49–60
© *1983 Alan R. Liss, Inc., 150 Fifth Avenue, New York, NY 10011*

UTILITY OF THE SKIN/UV-CARCINOGENESIS MODEL FOR EVALUATING THE ROLE OF NUTRITIONAL LIPIDS IN CANCER

Homer S. Black, Ph.D.

Photobiology Laboratory, Veterans Administration
Medical Center and Department of Dermatology,
Baylor College of Medicine, Houston, Texas 77211

INTRODUCTION

It is well documented that diet influences the rate of formation of certain types of chemically-induced and spontaneous tumors (Rusch 1944; Haven, Bloor 1956; Tannenbaum, Silverstone 1953, 1957; Carroll, Khor 1975; Clayson 1975; Vitale, 1975; Alcantara, Speckmann 1976; Visek et al 1978; Hayes, Campbell 1980). Lipids represent one particular class of dietary constituents thus implicated, the latter resulting from the early studies of Watson and Mellanby (1930) in which dietary fat was demonstrated to enhance coal tar-induced skin tumors and associated lung nodules. This effect of dietary fat upon chemical carcinogenesis was soon substantiated by others (Baumann, et al 1939; Tannenbaum 1942). Numerous studies have since been conducted of the quantitative and qualitative composition of dietary lipids and their relationship to tumor enhancement (Miller et al 1944; Carroll, Khor 1971, 1975; Carroll, Hopkins 1979). Miller et al (1944) reported that coconut oil, composed almost entirely of saturated lipids, would retard chemically-induced hepatomas in rats and suggested that unsaturated lipids might be necessary for development of those tumors. These workers reported that the inhibitory effect of coconut oil persisted when the animals were concurrently fed a high unsaturated fatty acid diet. Similarly, Carroll and Khor (1971) found that rats fed unsaturated lipids developed more mammary tumors than those fed the same levels of saturated lipids. More recently, however, studies from Carroll's laboratory (Carroll, Hopkins 1979) indicate that saturated fat enhances dimethylbenz(a)anthracene (DMBA)-induced mammary tumor yields as effectively as unsaturated fats when low levels of the latter are fed concurrently. These data indicate that, under the respective experimental conditions, a requirement for unsaturated lipid is manifested in both liver and mammmary carcinogenesis.

Epidemiologic evidence suggests that cancers of the digestive tract are also associated with dietary components (Weisburger et al 1977). Reddy (1981) has summarized the data relating dietary lipid to large bowel cancer in experimental animal models. He concludes that total level of dietary fat, more so than type, exerts a promoting effect upon chemically-induced carcinogenesis. However, here also, the data suggest a predisposition by unsaturated lipid on colon tumors induced with dimethylhydrazine (Broitman et al 1977; Reddy et al 1976). Definitive experiments remain to be conducted concerning unsaturated lipid requirements in digestive tract carcinogenesis. Nevertheless, there can be little doubt that dietary lipid, in general, can have a pronounced influence on the developmental course of several major forms of cancer.

LIPIDS AND PHOTOCARCINOGENESIS

Weisburger et al (1977) have reviewed the major research developments and epidemiologic evidence that support the contention that etiologies of the main human cancers stem largely from our life-styles. Whereas considerable evidence indicates that a large number of these cancers are associated with diet, especially diets containing high levels of fat, to our knowledge no epidemiological studies of diet and its relation to skin cancer have been reported. It is ironic that this potential relationship has received so little attention as, in this case, both the initiator of carcinogenesis (UV) and modifier (diet) so profoundly manifest life-style. There also seems to have been a lack of interest in diet and photocarcinogenesis, of an experimental nature, as the initial, and until recently the only, direct study of such a relationship was published in 1939 (Baumann, Rusch).

Cholesterol

Nearly 50 years ago A.H. Roffo (1933) suggested that cholesterol was involved in carcinogenesis, specifically actinic-induced cancer. He observed that individuals whose diets contained high cholesterol levels and whose activities resulted in excessive sun exposure were more subject to skin cancer. Further, he suggested that cholesterol was photo-oxidized to chemicals that were responsible for the carcinogenic properties of UV (Bergmann et al 1940). One such compound, the 5α, 6α-epoxide of cholesterol, was reported to be formed in human skin upon exposure to UV (Black, Lo 1971). It's role, if any, in the photocarcinogenic process remains obscure (Black, Chan 1976; Black 1980).

In order to test Roffo's theory that cholesterol in some way "prepares the soil" for the development of tumors, Baumann and Rusch (1939) conducted studies in which they evaluated the effects of dietary cholesterol on UV-induced skin cancer in albino mice. They reported that saturation of experimental animals with dietary cholesterol did not result in accelerated tumor formation.

Although a number of studies have since failed to demonstrate a relationship between cholesterol intake, serum cholesterol levels, and neoplasia (Wynder et al 1969; Westlund, Nicolaysen 1972; Howell 1975), the hypothesis that dietary cholesterol plays some role in tumor development has advanced on the basis of (1) epidemiological association between coronary artery disease and certain types of cancer (notably breast, colorectal, and some forms of adult leukemia) (Lea 1966; Rose et al 1974); (2) the elevated sterol synthetic levels associated with actively growing tissues and certain types of neoplasms, particularly the loss of feedback control of cholesterol biosynthesis associated with hepatoma (Siperstein, Fagan 1964; Sabine et al 1967; Horton, Sabine 1971); and (3) studies that demonstrate significantly lower serum cholesterol in patients with colon cancer (Bjelke 1974; Rose et al 1974). In at least one form of malignant transformation the evidence for cholesterol involvement is impressive. Inbar and Shinitzky (1974) have demonstrated that some forms of human and mammalian leukemia are accompanied by a marked deficiency of free cholesterol in the cell surface membranes. Concomitant with this deficiency, patients demonstrated both lowered blood cholesterol levels and hypocholesterolemia. The latter is associated with colon cancer as well.

The skin/UV model was employed to further examine the potential role of dietary cholesterol in carcinogenesis. Six hundred hairless mice (Skh-HR-1) were fed synthetic isocaloric diets containing either 2% (w/w) or no cholesterol (Black et al 1979). A regimen of escalating UV radiation was administered until a cumulative dose of 145 J/cm^2 had been delivered. Animals were evaluated for tumors, body weight, hematocrits, and serum cholesterol levels. A cumulative distribution frequency was used to determine tumor latency periods. The time for tumor development in 50% of the animals (TDT_{50}) receiving the high cholesterol diet was significantly longer than for those animals receiving no sterol (Figure 1). Although these data confirm the earlier observation of

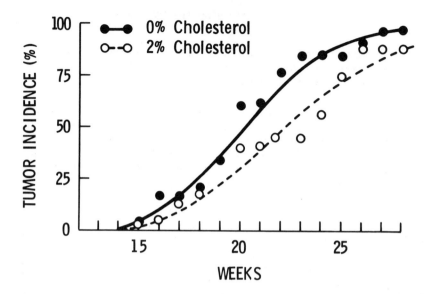

FIGURE 1. Effect of dietary cholesterol on the cumulative distribution of UV-induced tumor incidence. TDT_{50} values were 20.2 and 22.3 weeks for 0% and 2% dietary cholesterol levels respectively. Data taken from Black et al, 1979.

Baumann and Rusch (1939) in which cholesterol was found to have no enhancing effect upon the rate of UV-induced tumor formation, they indicate that dietary cholesterol has a slight, but significant, moderating effect. Whether this effect results from direct participation of cholesterol in the carcinogenic process or occurs as the result of sterol altered epidermal parameters that affect the dose of UV reaching respective target sites remains unknown. However, it appears certain that dietary sterol level is a nutritional factor capable of modifying the carcinogenic response to UV and thus should be carefully considered in future nutrition experiments.

Neutral Fats

Despite numerous experimental variables (e.g. radiation source, animal species, dietary caloric inequalities, etc.) that make comparisons with more recent studies impractical, Baumann and Rusch (1939) nevertheless were first to demonstrate that dietary lipid enhanced UV-carcinogenesis. By feeding a diet containing 30% hydrogenated cottonseed oil, they found a marked decrease in tumor development time.

In an effort to control nutritional parameters that otherwise would make interpretation of the results difficult, a study employing 500 hairless mice was initiated to access the influence of dietary lipid level and degree of lipid saturation upon photocarcinogenesis (Black et al In press). The animals received purified, isocaloric diets. As in the previous studies, a regimen of escalating UV radiation was employed and the animals were evaluated for tumors, hematocrits, and serum triglyceride levels. Although there were no significant differences in $TDT_{50}s$ between animals receiving low and high unsaturated dietary lipid regimens, animals receiving hydrogenated corn oil demonstrated a significantly longer TDT_{50} than in either 4% or 12% unsaturated lipid groups (Figure 2). Further, animals receiving hydrogenated corn oil exhibited fewer tumors per animal than those receiving either 4% or 12% of the unsaturated lipid. (Table 1). This apparent exacerbation of photocarcinogenesis by unsaturated lipid is not incompatible with the concept that these dietary constituents may be required just as indicated in certain cases of chemically-induced carcinogenesis (Carroll 1981).

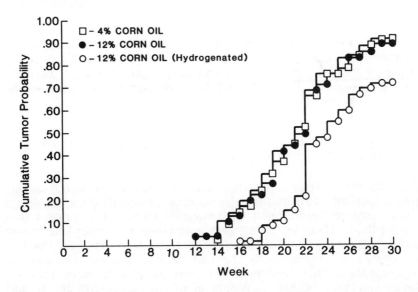

FIGURE 2. Life-table analysis of the effects of dietary lipid on UV-induced tumor probability. TDT_{50} values were 22.6, 22.9, and 26.3 weeks for 4%, 12%, and hydrogenated 12% corn oil respectively. Data taken from Black et al, in press.

MEAN NUMBER OF TUMORS PER ANIMAL

WEEK   TREATMENT GROUP

	1	2	3	4	5	6
25	2.78	3.06	3.17	5.67	1.12	1.21
26	2.97	3.58	2.90	6.18	1.29	1.00
27	3.91	4.76	4.07	6.91	1.27	1.64
28	3.82	5.34	3.70	6.52	1.45	1.42
29	4.41	5.48	3.68	6.94	1.20	1.38
30	4.97	6.00	4.79	7.15	2.31	2.19

Table 1. Effect of dietary lipid on UV-mediated tumor multiplicity. Treatment groups: 1, 4% corn oil; 2, 4% corn oil and antioxidants; 3, 12% corn oil; 4, 12% corn oil and antioxidants; 5, 12% corn oil (hydrogenated); 6, 12% corn oil (hydrogenated) and antioxidants. Data taken from Black et al, in press.

INTERACTION OF LIPIDS AND ANTIOXIDANTS: INFLUENCE UPON PHOTOCARCINOGENESIS

Whereas extreme caution must be exercised when making generalizations about dietary effects upon tumors of different origin and/or induced by different carcinogenic agents, it is evident that dietary lipid influences the carcinogenic process. Regardless, Rusch (1944) noted major differences, aside from fatty acid composition and degree of saturation, in the various lipid sources employed in experiments of that era. Notable among those differences were the the antioxidant properties. A number of chemicals with antioxidant properties have now been shown to modify the effects of chemical carcinogens (Wattenberg 1972, 1975). Similar effects by antioxidants upon photocarcinogenesis have also been reported (Black 1974; Black et al 1978). The prospect of a relationship between dietary lipid, antioxidants, and interactions which may influence carcinogenesis is beginning to emerge.

Accordingly, we have observed that unsaturated lipid, at 4% or 12% of the diet, and antioxidants interact to increase tumor multiplicity (Table 1). Our previous studies had demonstrated a significant reduction in UV-induced tumor development when animals were fed a closed formula commercial ration supplemented with antioxidants. However, we noted that the magnitude of this salutary response was diminished when the antioxidants were supplied in defined diets containing 2% corn oil as lipid source (Black et al 1979). In earlier studies we had supplemented animals with a mixture of antioxidants, including ascorbic acid, dl-α-tocopherol, reduced glutathione, and butylated hydroxytoluene (BHT). All, except BHT, were ineffective in inhibiting UV-induced tumor formation when tested individually at concentrations comparable to those used in mixture (Black et al 1978; Pauling et al In press). Therefore BHT is assumed to be the active principal contained in the mixture. In this regard, King et al (1979) have reported that dietary unsaturated lipid acts antagonistically to BHT, resulting in a higher incidence of DMBA-induced mammary tumors compared to animals fed comparable diets containing saturated lipid and BHT. Studies by McCay et al (1980) indicate that unsaturated dietary fat promotes the growth of established tumor cell clones, ie tumor promotion, although some events involved in initiation may also be affected.

The basis for selecting antioxidants as potential chemopreventive agents stems from their ability to scavenge detrimental free radicals or terminate chain reactions initiated by them. Demopoulos et al (1980) have discussed the potential of dietary polyunsaturated fatty acids to alter membrane characteristics and accelerate free radical reactions. Studies from Carroll's laboratory, and those of McCay et al, have shown that (1) dietary polyunsaturates enhance carcinogenesis and subsequent tumor growth and (2) that antioxidants can ameliorate the effects of dietary unsaturated lipid. These observations indirectly support the hypothesis that free radical reactions are, in some manner, involved in the carcinogenic process. Free radicals have been reported to be formed in UV-radiated skin as well (Pathak, Stratton 1968). However, in our recent studies we found not just an antagonistic interaction between unsaturated fat and antioxidants, as would be expected by antioxidant quenching of free radical reactions initiated by unsaturates, but rather an exacerbation by antioxidants upon unsaturated lipid-enhanced photocarcinogenesis. The influence of unsaturated lipid-antioxidant interactions upon photocarcinogenesis is summarized in Table 2. These data indicate that antioxidants, in the presence of low levels of unsaturated lipid, have an inhibitory

Lipid Level	Tumor Latency TDT$_{50}$ (Days) AO+ vs AO-	Tumor Multiplicity Tumors/animal (AO+/AO- ratio)
2%	+ 28.5	0.52
4%	- 2.5	1.10
12%	- 16.2	1.79

TABLE 2. Effects of unsaturated lipid-antioxidant interactions on photocarcinogenesis. 25 week data from two comparable studies. AO, antioxidants.

effect upon photocarcinogenesis in terms of both tumor latency period and multiplicity. However, as the level of unsaturated lipid is increased, the chemopreventive effects of antioxidants are not only negated but enhancement of photocarcinogenesis ultimately occurs. In an attempt to explain these findings we have suggested that antioxidants alter host metabolism in a manner that allows maximum expression of unsaturated lipid-enhanced tumorigenesis. This effect is probably expressed at the promotional stage of tumor development. This could account for the increased tumor multiplicity observed in animals receiving both unsaturated lipid and antioxidant supplements. That antioxidants and unsaturated lipid have the capability of altering hepatic capacity for carcinogen metabolism has recently been demonstrated (Black, Gerguis 1980). Whether similar alterations of cutaneous metabolism occur is unknown.

CONCLUSIONS:

Previous studies of the influence of dietary lipids on photocarcinogenesis have shown that: (1) tumor latency time in animals receiving high dietary levels of cholesterol is significantly increased, (2) tumor latency time in animals receiving unsaturated lipid was significantly less than that of animals fed saturated lipid, (3) Tumor multiplicity in animals fed saturated lipid was significantly less than that which occurred in those animals fed unsaturated lipid, and (4) certain levels of unsaturated lipids and antioxidants interact to increase tumor multiplicity and decrease tumor latency periods. These data not only underscore the similarities of response induced by dietary lipid to both UV and chemical carcinogens but suggest a general participation of lipids in the carcinogenic process. If that role occurs at the promotional stage of carcinogenesis, then dietary modification could prove beneficial in both prevention and management of actinic skin cancer—a disease with a great propensity for repeated tumor occurrence.

Not only do similarities of response occur between chemical and UV mediated carcinogenesis but the skin/UV-carcinogenesis model appears to be equally sensitive to dietary modification. Thus it should prove useful in evaluating the role of dietary lipids in cancer. In addition, the skin/UV model provides some unique advantages for the evaluation of carcinogenesis inhibitors as well as insight to their interactions with lipids. In UV-carcinogenesis no activation or detoxification of the presumed carcinogenic species is involved as is the case with chemical carcinogenesis. No competitive chemical inhibition occurs nor does transport of carcinogen to respective target sites complicate the response. UV is a complete carcinogen to the epidermis and it can be delivered quantitatively to the target tissue. The end result of UV radiation can be easily visualized and quantitated. With due consideration to other experimental parameters, the skin/UV model should prove valuable in evaluating the efficacy of potential anticarcinogenic agents, elucidating their modes of action, and determining the nature of their interactions with dietary lipid.

ACKNOWLEDGEMENTS

The author's work was supported in part by PHS grant CA-20907 from the NCI.

REFERENCES

Alcantara EN, Speckmann EW (1976). Diet, nutrition, and cancer. Am J Clin Nutr 29:1035.

Baumann CA, Jacobi HP, Rusch HP (1939). The effect of diet on experimental tumor production. Am J Hyg 30:1.

Baumann CA, Rusch HP (1939). Effect of diet on tumors induced by ultra-violet light. Am J Cancer 35:213.

Bergmann W, Stavely HE, Strong LC, Smith GM (1940). Studies on the hypothetical carcinogenecity of irradiated sterols. I. The effects of irradiated cholesterol on the skin of mice. Am J Cancer 38:81.

Bjelke E (1974). Colon cancer and blood-cholesterol. Lancet 1:1116.

Black HS (1974). Effects of dietary antioxidants on actinic tumor induction. Res Commun Chem Path Pharmacol 7:783

Black HS (1980). Analysis and physiologic significance of cholesterol epoxide in animals tissues. Lipids 15: 705.

Black HS, Chan JT (1976). Etiologic related studies of UVL-mediated carcinogenesis. Oncology 33:119.

Black HS, Chan JT, Brown GE (1978). Effects of dietary constituents on ultraviolet light-mediated carcinogenesis. Cancer Res 38:1384.

Black HS, Gerguis J (1980). Use of the Ames test in assessing the relation of dietary lipid and antioxidants to N-2-Fluorenylacetamide activation. J Environ Path Toxicol 4:131.

Black HS, Henderson SV, Kleinhans CM, Phelps AW, Thornby JI (1979). Effect of dietary cholesterol on ultraviolet light carcinogenesis. Cancer Res 39:5022.

Black HS, Lenger W, Phelps AW, Thornby JI (In press). Influence of dietary lipid upon ultraviolet light-carcinogenesis. J Environ Path Toxicol.

Black HS, Lo WB (1971). Formation of a carcinogen in UV-irradiated human skin. Nature 234:306.

Broitman SA, Vitale JJ, Vavrousek-Jakuba E, Gottlieb LS (1977). Polysaturated fat, cholesterol and large bowel tumorigenesis. Cancer 40:2455.

Carroll KK (1981). Neutral fats and cancer. Cancer Res 41:3695.

Carroll KK, Hopkins GT (1979). Dietary polyunsaturated fat versus saturated fat in relation to mammary carcinogenesis. Lipids 14:155.

Carroll KK, Khor HT (1971). Effects of level and type of dietary fat on the incidence of mammary tumors induced in female Sprague-Dawley rats by 7,12-dimethylbenz(a) anthracene. Lipids 6:415.

Carroll KK, Khor HT (1975). Dietary fat in relation to tumorigenesis. Progr Biochem Pharmacol 10:308.

Clayson DB (1975). Nutrition and experimental carcinogenesis: A review. Cancer Res 35:3292.

Demopoulos HB, Pietronigro DD, Flamm ES, Seligman ML (1980). The possible role of free radical reactions in carcinogenesis. J Environ Path Toxicol 3:273.

Haven FL, Bloor WR (1956). Lipids in cancer. Adv Cancer Res 4:237.

Hayes JR, Campbell TC (1980). Nutrition as a modifier of chemical carcinogenesis. In Slaga TJ (ed). "Carcinogenesis: Modifiers of Chemical Carcinogenesis", Vol 5, Raven Press, N.Y., p 207.

Horton BJ, Sabine JR (1971). Metabolic controls in precancerous liver: defective control of cholesterol synthesis in rats fed N-2-fluorenylacetamide. Eur J Cancer 7:459.

Howell MA (1975). Diet as an etiologic factor in the development of cancers of the colon and rectum. J Chronic Dis 28:67.

Inbar M, Shinitzky M (1974). Cholesterol as a bioregulator in the development and inhibition of leukemia. Proc Natl Acad Sci USA 71:4229.

King MM, Bailey DM, Gibson DD, Pitha JV, McCay PB (1979).Incidence and growth of mammary tumors induced by 7, 12-dimethybenz(a)anthracene as related to the dietary content of fat and antioxidant. J Natl Cancer Inst 63:657.

Lea AJ (1966). Dietary factors associated with death-rates from certain neoplasms in man. Lancet 2:332.

McCay PB, King M, Rikans LE, Pitha JV (1980). Interactions between dietary fats and antioxidants on DMBA-induced mammary carcinomas and on AAF-induced hyperplastic nodules and hepatomas. J Environ Path Toxicol 3:451.

Pathak MA, Stratton K (1968). Free radicals in human skin before and after exposure to light. Arch Biochem Biophys 123:468.

Pauling L, Willoughby R, Reynolds R, Blaisdell BE, Lawson S (In press). Incidence of squamous cell carcinonoma in hairless mice irradiated with ultraviolet light in relation to intake of ascorbic acid (vitamin C) and of D,L-α- tocopheryl acetate (vitamin E). Proc. Third Internat. Symposium on Vitamin C, Sao Paulo, Brazil.

Reddy BS (1981). Dietary fat and its relationship to large bowel cancer. Cancer Res 41:3700.

Reddy BS, Narisawa T, Vukusich D, Weisburger JH, Wynder EL (1976). Effect of quality and quantity of dietary fat and dimethylhydrazine in colon carcinogenesis of rats. Proc Soc Exp Biol Med 151:237.

Roffo AH (1933). Heliotropism of cholesterol in relation to skin cancer. Am J Cancer 17:42.

Rose G, Blackburn H, Keys A, Taylor HL, Kannel WB, Paul O, Reid DD, Stamler J (1974). Colon cancer and blood cholesterol. Lancet 1:181.

Rusch HP (1944). Extrinsic factors that influence carcinogenesis. Physiol Rev 24:177.

Sabine JR, Abraham S, Chaikoff IL (1967). Control of lipid metabolism in hepatomas: insensitivity of rate of fatty acid and cholesterol synthesis by mouse hepatoma BW7756 to fasting and to feedback control. Cancer Res 27:793.

Siperstein MD, Fagan VM (1964). Studies on the feed-back regulation of cholesterol synthesis. Adv Enzyme Regul 2:249.

Tannenbaum A (1942). The genesis and growth of tumors, III. Effects of a high-fat diet. Cancer Res 2:468.

Tannenbaum A, Silverstone H (1953). Nutrition in relation to cancer. Adv Cancer Res 1:451.

Tannenbaum A, Silverstone H (1957). Nutrition and genesis of tumors. In Raven, RW (ed): "Cancer", Vol 1, London: Butterworth, p. 306.

Visek WJ, Clinton SK, Truex CR (1978). Nutrition and experimental carcinogenesis. The Cornell Veterinarian 68:3.

Vitale JJ (1975). Possible role of nutrients in neoplasia. Cancer Res 35:3320.

Watson AF, Mellanby E (1930). Tar cancer in mice, II. The condition of the skin when modified by external treatment or diet, as a factor in influencing this cancerous reaction. Brit J Exptl Path 11:311.

Wattenberg LW (1972). Inhibition of carcinogenic and toxic effects of polycyclic hydrocarbons by phenolic antioxidants and ethoxyquin. J Natl Cancer Inst 48:1425.

Wattenberg LW (1975). Effects of dietary constituents on the metabolism of chemical carcinogens. Cancer Res 35:3326.

Weisburger JH, Cohen LA, Wynder EL (1977). On the etiology and metabolic epidemiology of the main human cancers. In Hiatt HH, Watson JD, Winsten JA (eds): "Origins of Human Cancer", Vol A , Cold Spring Harbor Laboratory, p 567.

Westlund K, Nicolaysen R (1972). Ten-year mortality and morbidity related to serum cholesterol. Scand J Clin Lab Invest 30 (Suppl. 127):1.

Wynder EL, Kajitani T, Ishikawa S, Dodo H, Takano A (1969). Environmental factors of cancer of the colon and rectum. Cancer Res 23:1210.

Diet, Nutrition, and Cancer:
From Basic Research to Policy Implications, pages 61–90
© *1983 Alan R. Liss, Inc., 150 Fifth Avenue, New York, NY 10011*

DIETARY FAT MAY INFLUENCE DMBA-INITIATED MAMMARY GLAND
CARCINOGENESIS BY MODIFICATION OF MAMMARY GLAND
DEVELOPMENT

M. Margaret King, Ph.D. [1], Paul B. McCay, Ph.D. [1],
and Irma H. Russo, M.D. [2]

[1]Biomembrane Research Laboratory
Oklahoma Medical Research Foundation, and
Department of Biochemistry and Molecular
  Biology
University of Oklahoma Health Sciences Center
Oklahoma City, Oklahoma 73104

[2]Experimental Pathology Laborabory
Department of Biology
Michigan Cancer Foundation
Detroit, Michigan 48201

The influence of the type and amount of dietary fat
on DMBA-induced rat mammary gland tumor incidence and
tumor growth rate, as well as the effect of dietary antioxidants is under investigation in our laboratory under
conditions of controlled dietary composition. The rationale for pursuing this series of experiments was as follows. As information on the nutritional requirements of
various animal species unfolded over the years, it became
established that the intake of elevated levels of dietary
fat, particularly polyunsaturated fat must be accompanied
by an elevated level of dietary antioxidant (Horwitt
1970). If such an antioxidant were lacking, animals consuming such diets exhibited various pathological, somewhat
species-specific tissue damage (Dam 1957). The higher the
polyunsaturated fatty acid intake, the higher the antioxidant requirement became in order to prevent such damage.
The elucidation of α-tocopherol as vitamin E developed
from such studies since it was determined to be the effective naturally occuring antioxidant which provided protection to tissues from the damaging effect of polyunsatu-

rated fat-feeding (Witting 1969). It was soon found that other, structurally unrelated antioxidants could afford similar protection against the injurious effects of unsaturated fat consumption (Vasington, Reichard, Nason 1960). Furthermore, it was demonstrated by Bieri and coworkers that some species fed very low dietary fat levels had no apparent requirement for an antioxidant at all (Bieri, Briggs, Pollard, Spivey-Fox 1960). Some dietary polyunsaturated fat is essential for life in higher organisms since the total polyunsaturated fatty acid structure required for prostaglandin synthesis cannot be synthesized in those organisms. Hence, the requirement for linoleic acid to be provided in the diet (Mohrhauer, Holman 1963). This fatty acid originates in the food chain from a variety of plant sources (Aaes-Jorgensen 1961). Nevertheless, an intake of linoleic acid at the normal intake level of most Americans would result in extensive tissue damage to certain organs in laboratory animals (especially young, rapidly developing animals) unless an adequate intake of dietary antioxidant accompanied the fat consumed. The lesions produced almost always include development of necrotic foci in the affected tissues, which can ultimately lead to loss of function of the organ(s) in which this tissue is an integral part. If the organ affected in a given species is a vital one, the animal dies. Hence rabbits (Draper, Csallany 1958), rats (Schwarz 1952), fowl (Pappenheimer, Goetsch 1931), etc., perish within a relatively short period of time when fed an antioxidant-deficient diet rich in polyunsaturated fat during the postweaning (or post-hatching) period of rapid development. In spite of intensive investigations to determine the mechanism of this highly reproducible effect, the mechanism of the tissue injury still remains elusive, although peroxidative alterations of membrane lipids are strongly implicated in the etiology (Witting 1979).

The apparent antagonistic effect of dietary unsaturated fat and dietary antioxidant, as well as the separate observations indicating that dietary fat enhanced tumorigenesis (Carroll 1975) while antioxidants decreased it (Wattenberg 1978), led us to investigate the relationship between dietary fat unsaturation levels and dietary antioxidants as a function of their influence on mammary gland carcinogenesis. World-wide epidemiological surveys have generated data showing a significant correlation between the per capita consumption of dietary fat and the incidence of mammary and colon cancer in those regions (Wynder 1976). The U.S. has one of the highest per capita consumption levels of fat in the world and also rates amoung the highest in the incidence of cancer of the colon and mammary gland. Hence, the use of animal models in which mammary and colon carcinogenesis is similarly enhanced by dietary fat should be extremely valuable in the search for mechanisms.

The antagonism between dietary fats and antioxidants on carcinogenesis caused by a variety of agents suggests that a common factor may be involved in the balance between dietary unsaturated fat and antioxidant content required to maintain tissue integrity. The common factor may be lipid peroxidation. There is a considerable body of evidence indicating that lipid peroxidation occurs at an accelerated rate in animals fed diets rich in polyunsaturated fat but low in antioxidant (Witting 1969). Arguments have been mounted that the accelerated accumulation of lipofuscin pigments in brain, heart, testes, and muscle in animals fed elevated levels of unsaturated fats without increased levels of antioxidant is a consequence of lipid peroxidation (Norkin 1966). Because lipid peroxides are strong oxidants, they are known to be capable of interacting with carcinogens, particularly lipid-soluble ones, or their metabolites, to produce products which may influence tumorigenesis. An example of the possible role of peroxidic compounds may be the promotional effect of benzoyl peroxide on skin tumorigenesis initiated by 7,12-dimethylbenz(α)anthracene (Slaga, Klein-Syanto, Triplett, Yotti, Trosko 1981).

Our approach to the relationship between dietary fats and antioxidants to carcinogenesis was to investigate 1) how the level of fat unsaturation per se influenced the capacity of antioxidants to inhibit mammary gland tumorigenesis; 2) the effect of the time during which the antioxidant to be tested is supplied to the animal with respect to the time at which the single dose of DMBA is administered; and 3) the effect of the diets which were used in these studies on the developmental state of the mammary gland at the time of carcinogen exposure.

1.   THE INFLUENCE OF THE AMOUNT AND DEGREE OF UNSATURA-
TION OF DIETARY FAT ON THE CAPACITY OF ANTIOXIDANTS TO
INHIBIT MAMMARY CARCINOGENESIS.

The observation that dietary fat levels enhanced
mammary carcinogenesis by DMBA was made more than a decade
ago by Carroll and co-workers (Carroll, Gammal, Plunkett
1968; Gammal, Carroll, Plunkett 1967). These workers
reported that mammary tumor incidence following DMBA administration was increased by raising fat levels in the
diet and that the more unsaturated the fat, the higher the
tumor yield. Enhancement of the incidence of other types
of tumors including "spontaneous" ones associated with
raising dietary fat content has also been reported
(Benson, Lev, Grand 1956; Engel, Copeland 1951;
Silverstone, Tannenbaum 1950). This effect of dietary fat
on tumor incidence is now well-established, but the mechanisms of this phenomenon is not known. The effect is not
a consequence of differences in caloric densities of the
diets fed (Chan, Dao 1981; Engel, Copeland 1951;
Tannenbaum 1945), but rather one which appears to be truly
related to the type and amount of fat in the diet.

Three basic diets were employed in the studies performed in our laboratory: a low-fat diet (2% linoleic
acid) and two high-fat diets. One of the latter contained
highly polyunsaturated fat (20% stripped corn oil) while
the other contained the same amount of total fat but was
mostly saturated (18% hydrogenated coconut oil plus 2%
linoleic acid). All of these diets contained adequate
levels of essential fatty acids for the young, growing
rat. The complete composition of these diets is shown in
Table 1. Note that the amount of unsaturated fat in the
low-fat diet and the saturated high-fat diet are the same.
The same diets were prepared in which one of the following
antioxidants was supplemented at the indicated level: α-
tocopherol, 0.2%; butylated hydroxytoluene, 0.3%; butylated hydroxyanisole, 0.3% and propyl gallate, 0.3%.
Groups of weanling (21 day-old) female, Sprague-Dawley
rats were fed one of these diets throughout the period of
the experiment. At 50 days of age, the rats were given a
single dose of 7,12-dimethylbenz(α)anthracene dissolved in
stripped corn oil by intragastric intubation. From 10-11
weeks of age onward, the rats were monitored at least
once each week for weight gain and mammary tumor development. Weight gain was essentially identical in all

EXPERIMENTAL DIETS

	HIGH POLYUNSATURATED FAT DIET	HIGH SATURATED FAT DIET	LOW FAT DIET
	% BY WT.	% BY WT.	% BY WT.
CASEIN	23	23	23
FAT	20 [a]	20 [b]	2 [c]
SUCROSE	46	46	64
SALT MIXTURE [d]	4	4	4
ALPHACEL (NON-NUTRIENT BULK	6	6	6
VITAMIN MIXTURE [e]	1	1	1

[a] STRIPPED CORN OIL

[b] 18% COCONUT OIL + 2% LINOLEIC ACID METHYL ESTERS

[c] 2% LINOLEIC ACID METHYL ESTERS

[d] AIN -76 MINERAL MIXTURE

[e] AIN -76 VITAMIN MIXTURE

dietary groups, both with and without antioxidant supplementation. Tumor incidence results are shown in Fig. 1. It is immediately apparent that there is a marked difference in tumor incidence between rats fed the three basal diets. The animals fed the low fat diet had less than half the tumor incidence of those fed the polyunsaturated fat diet, while the incidence in the saturated fat diet-fed animals was about 70% of the unsaturated fat diet group. Both the saturated fat diet and the low fat diet had the same amount of essential fatty acid per gram of diet, but the saturated fat diet contained 10 times the amount of total fat as the low-fat diet. However, the amount of fat in the unsaturated and the saturated fat diets was identical, and this clearly shows that the degree of unsaturation has a significant influence on tumor incidence.

DIETARY FAT AND ANTIOXIDANT INFLUENCES ON DMBA-INDUCED MAMMARY CARCINOGENESIS

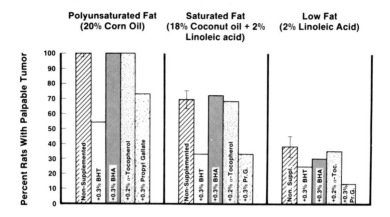

Fig. 1: Mammary tumor incidence in female Sprague-Dawley rats at 30 weeks of age. Unsupplemented dietary control groups were paired with each antioxidant group (thus being expressed + S.E. of 4 separate experiments). Diets were as described in Table 1 (N = 30).

A second readily apparent feature of the data in Fig. 1 is that while feeding of diets supplemented with BHT and propyl gallate both inhibited tumorigenesis in animals fed any of the three basal diets, neither α-tocopherol nor butylated hydroxyanisole supplementation had an influence on the incidence of tumors. This differential effect of these antioxidants has been verified in subsequent experiments using both purified diets and by simply adding the antioxidant to pulverized commercial laboratory rat ration. Since both BHA and α-tocopherol are good antioxidants, the data suggests that antioxidants as a class of compounds are not inhibitors of carcinogenesis, but certain antioxidants do inhibit significantly.

In considering the possible reasons why BHT and propyl gallate decreased mammary incidence significantly while BHA and α-tocopherol had no effect, properties other than that of inhibition of oxidation were considered. BHT induces hepatic cytochrome P-450, a component of the microsomal mixed function oxidase system (King, McCay 1981). Both BHT and propyl gallate, on the other hand, induce microsomal epoxide hydratase (unpublished observation). α-Tocopherol and BHA, however, had no noticeable effect on cytochrome P-450 content at the supplementation levels given. Since DMBA is known to require metabolic activation in order to initiate carcinogenesis (Kinoshita, Gelboin 1972), these observations suggest that changes in the metabolism of DMBA by BHT resulting in modification of the mixed function oxidase system might be responsible for the inhibitory effect of these two antioxidants on tumorigenesis. If that were the case, the results obtained in Fig. 1 could be explained.

To obtain further insight into the possibility that BHT and propyl gallate were modifying carcinogen metabolism in animals supplemented with those antioxidants, the influence of BHT on mammary tumor formation in female rats treated with nitrosomethylurea (NMU) was tested. NMU is a direct-acting carcinogen (Richards, Nandi 1978), not requiring metabolic activivation. Hence, if BHT were acting by modifying the activation of carcinogens, one would not expect supplementation of the diet with this antioxidant to modify tumorigenesis caused by NMU. Fig. 2 shows that BHT feeding to animals given a single dose of NMU had no significant influence on mammary tumor incidence. The level of BHT given was the same (0.3%) as that which resulted in significant inhibition of DMBA-induced rat mammary gland tumorigenesis . These results give further support to the hypothesis that BHT may be inhibiting carcinogenesis by altering the activation of carcinogens requiring this metabolic reaction.

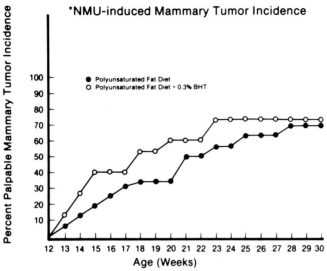

*NMU-induced Mammary Tumor Incidence

● Polyunsaturated Fat Diet
○ Polyunsaturated Fat Diet + 0.3% BHT

NMU = N-nitrosomethylurea single i.v. dose as 50 mg/kg body wt. at 50 days of age
BHT = Butylated hydroxytoluene added to the diet at 0.3% by weight.

Fig. 2: Mammary tumor incidence in female Sprague-Dawley rats at 30 weeks of age. At 50 days of age the animals were treated with 5 mg nitrosomethylurea/100 g body wt i.v. via the tail vein and monitored for mammary tumor development.

2. THE EFFECT OF THE TIME OF BHT ADMINISTRATION ON DMBA-INDUCED MAMMARY CARCINOGENESIS.

In an effort to determine the critical time during which the antioxidant BHT must be fed to the animal to obtain protection against DMBA induced mammary carcinogenesis, the time and duration of feeding was varied with respect to carcinogen administration. Based on our previous tumor incidence studies, it was decided that only the two high-fat diets (20% stripped corn oil, and 18% coconut oil + 2% linoleic acid) would be utilized in these studies. The cumulative tumor incidence in the low-fat-fed group was not likely to yield significant differences, since this incidence is routinely low (i.e. 30-40% see Fig. 1), even without the inclusion of BHT. Manipulation of such a narrow range was not felt to be meaningful. Otherwise the experimental protocol utilized a single 10 mg dose of DMBA at 50 days of age and was identical to that used in previous incidence studies.

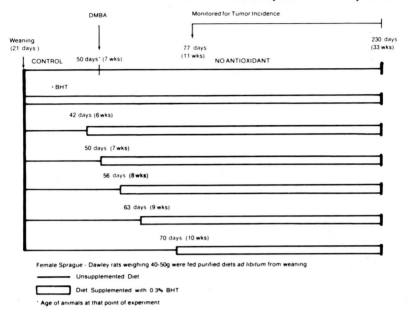

Fig. 3: Experimental protocol for BHT Timed-Study I. BHT (0.3% by wt) was added to either the high polyunsaturated diet or the high saturated fat diet at the various times as indicated and maintained in the diet throughout the experimental period (30 weeks of age). N = 30/group/time period.

Two separate and complimentary studies were performed. In the first approach to the investigation of the effectiveness of BHT with respect to time (BHT Timed-Study I), BHT feeding was initiated at times ranging from four weeks prior to carcinogen administration up to three weeks following carcinogen exposure (see Fig. 3 for the experimental design). In this experiment, once the BHT was added to the diet, it was maintained as a dietary additive throughout the remainder of the study, i.e. until the animals were 30 weeks of age. In a parallel experiment (BHT Timed-Study II) (Fig. 4), BHT was added to the diet for only short periods of time, varying the initiation of the supplementation by weekly intervals. The times of BHT addition were as follows: BHT added to diet at weaning (designated as zero time) and continuing the feeding for one of the following; 1 week, 2 weeks, 3 weeks, 4 weeks

(time of DMBA exposure) etc., up to 8 weeks from the
time of weaning (See Fig. 3). The BHT was then removed
from the diet at the times indicated, but the animals
continued to be maintained on their respective non-BHT
supplemented semi-purified diets for the remainder of the
experiment (33 weeks of age).

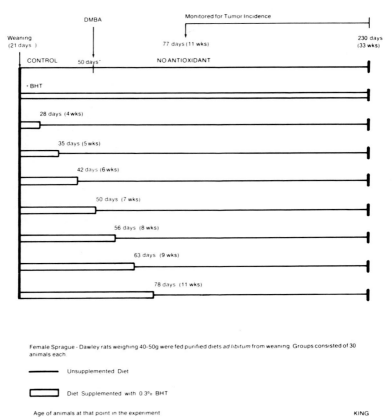

Fig. 4: Experimental protocol for BHT Timed-Study II.
BHT (0.3% by wt) was added to either the high polyunsaturated or the high saturated fat diets for only short time
intervals prior to and just after DMBA (10 mg i.g. at 50
days of age) treatment as indicated. N = 30/group/time
period.

BHT-Timed Study I

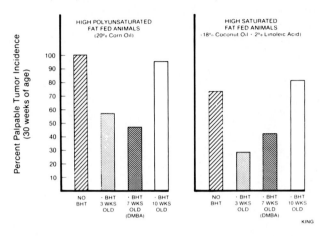

Fig. 5: Experimental results of BHT Timed-Study I. Mammary tumor incidence at 30 weeks of age in animals consuming high fat diets + BHT as indicated below bars.

Fig. 5 shows that BHT was effective in reducing tumor development when added to the diet just before and up to the time of DMBA exposure. The effectiveness of BHT in inhibiting tumorigenesis decreased as the time of initiating BHT feeding after carcinogen treatment increased. When BHT feeding was initiated three weeks post-DMBA treatment, it had no influence on mammary tumor development. The results indicate that the time for BHT to be most effective as an inhibitor of DMBA-induced tumorigenesis is during the three week period immediately preceding carcinogen exposure. Similar results were obtained in both the high polyunsaturated and high saturated fat-fed dietary groups, subsequently, in the BHT-Timed Study II, BHT was added to the diet for only short periods after weaning, ranging from 1 week (28 days of age) to 7 weeks (70 days of age). Fig. 5 shows that animals fed either of the high fat diets were afforded some protection (10-15% decrease in tumor incidence) when given BHT for three weeks after weaning (1 week prior to DMBA treatment).

This protection increased (approximately 20% inhibition) if BHT was left in the diet up to the time of carcinogen administration (4 weeks of BHT supplementation), but was maximal if continued until 1, 2 or 3 weeks after DMBA administration (40-50% inhibition of tumor incidence)- (Figs. 6&7).

These combined results indicate that the most crucial period of time for BHT to be present in the diet ranges somewhere between 1-2 weeks prior to the time of carcinogen exposure, up to 3 weeks after DMBA treatment. This suggests that BHT may be influencing the metabolic activation of DMBA, the initiation phase, or early promotional events associated with the DMBA exposure. Additional investigation may permit a more definitive description for the mechanism of the inhibition of DMBA-induced mammary carcinogenesis.

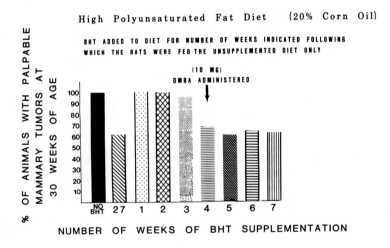

Fig. 6: Mammary tumor incidence in female Sprague-Dawley rats consuming diets + BHT (0.3% by wt) for the time intervals indicated below the bars. Past this time and until the end of the study (30 weeks of age) they consumed the high polyunsaturated diet with BHT supplementation.

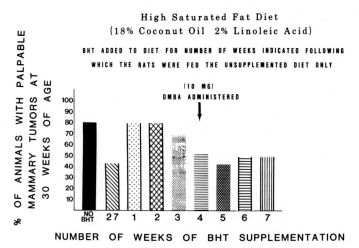

Fig. 7: Mammary tumor incidence in female Sprague-Dawley rats consuming a high saturated fat diet supplemented with 0.3% BHT for only the period of time indicated below the bars. Past this time and until the end of the study (30 weeks of age) they consumed the same diet without BHT supplementation.

3. THE EFFECT OF DIETARY FAT AND OF BHT SUPPLEMENTATION ON MAMMARY GLAND DEVELOPMENT

Recognition that nutritional factors, especially dietary fat, can have a profound influence on the susceptibility of individuals to carcinogenesis makes it imperative that an understanding of the mechanisms involved be determined. Both epidemiological and animal experimentation studies have indicated that dietary factors may be important in altering the response of individuals to environmental carcinogens. The epidemiological studies have indicated that breast cancer risk in the human female population is directly and positively correlated with nulliparity, increased age at first full-term pregnancy, and early onset of menses (Juret, Couette, Mandard,

Carre, Delozier, Brune, Vernhes 1976;   MacMahon, Cole,
Brown 1973).   While an early pregnancy seems to reduce the
risk of developing breast cancer (MacMahon, Cole, Brown
1973; MacMahon, Cole, Lin, Lowe, Mirra, Ravinihar, Salber,
Valaoras, Yvasa 1970), other studies have suggested that
there may be a difference in the extent to which height
and weight may operate as risk factors (Craig, Comstock,
Geisen 1974).   It is possible that at least some of these
factors may operate as indicators of nutritional effects.

Additionally, breast tissue appears to be more sensitive to such factors as ionizing radiation when exposure
occurs between 15 and 19 years of age, as was noted in the
Japanese population (Boice, Monson 1977;   McGregor, Land,
Choi, Tokjoka, Lui, Wakabayashie, Beebe 1977).   This implies that events occuring during the earlier years of
life in the human female may have a significant effect on
the lifetime risk of breast cancer.

An understanding of these mechanisms that make the
mammary glands of young women more susceptible to the
carcinogenic process has been explored by means of an
experimental rat model system.   As described above, this
system utilizes the rapid and reproducible induction of
mammary adenocarcinomas in the female Sprague-Dawley rat
by administration of the carcinogen (DMBA)(Dao 1964;
Huggins, Grand, Brillantes 1967).   This model mimics the
most significant features of the human disease (Moon 1969;
Russo, Russo, Ireland, Saby 1967; Russo, Saby, Isenberg,
Russo 1977) in that: the tumors are similar histologically to human breast tumors (Dao 1964;   Murad, von Haam
1972; Russo, Saby, Isenberg, Russo 1977);   they occur with
a high frequency in nulliparous rats (Huggins, Grand,
Brillantes 1959; Russo, Russo, Ireland, Saby 1977);   tumor
growth is stimulated by pregnancy, but full-term pregnancy
and lactation prior to carcinogen administration inhibits
tumor development (Moon 1969; MacMahon, Cole, Brown 1973;
Russo and Russo 1978a).   Thus, observations in the human,
as well as similar observations in murine models, suggest
that the degree of differentiation of the mammary gland at
the time of exposure to an etiologic agent may be very
important in the initiation of carcinogenesis.

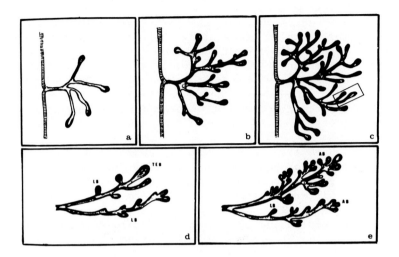

Fig. 8: Diagrammatic representation of the postnatal development of the female rat mammary gland: a) first week; b) second week; c) third week; d) details of the inset in c showing the TEB and lateral bud (LB); e) TEB differentiated into smaller structures called AB. Reprinted by permission from: (Russo and Russo 1978b).

Postnatal development of the rat mammary gland has been described by a number of investigators (Astwood, Geschickter, Rausch 1937; Russo, Russo 1978, a and b; Russo, Russo, Ireland, Saby 1977). Russo et al. (Russo, Saby, Isenberg, Russo 1977) found that at birth and during the first week of life the gland is composed of a single main lactiferous duct that branches into 3-5 narrow, straight secondary ducts (Fig. 8). These ducts end in small club-shaped terminal end buds (TEB). Sprouting of the ducts continues until the density of TEB (TEB/mm) reaches a maximum at 3 weeks of age, resulting in a corresponding increase in total area of the gland. From 3-10 weeks of age the TEB and lateral buds undergo a process of septation and cleavage to form alveolar buds (AB), starting from the nipple area and progressing peripherally. AB increase steadily as TEB decrease, until around 84 days of age, after which time the AB's remain almost constant in virgin rats. After the beginning of estrus at 35-42 days of age, lobular development begins. Lobular density increases progressively until approximately 10 weeks of age, after which it plateaus and remains constant as long as the animal is a virgin. A large number of TEB never differentiate in the virgin, but instead decrease in size due to hypoplasia of the epithelium, resulting in terminal ducts (TD). TD density increases, with age, but plateaus by 10-12 weeks and does not undergo further morphologic change.

Russo et al., (Russo, Wilgus, Russo 1979) found that at 45-55 days of age (the optimum time for DMBA administration to result in 100% tumor incidence) the TEB were actively differentiating into AB and had a high DNA labeling index (Fig. 9). Glands of older virgin rats, having fewer TEB and TD and fewer labeled cells, developed fewer carcinomas (63%). Glands of multiparous rats contained no TEB, only a few TD and very few labeled cells. DMBA administration to these rats resulted in a very low incidence of carcinomas (21%). Through careful correlations of structural development and DNA labeling indices with the age at time of carcinogen exposure and resulting neoplasias, they were able to relate density of TEB, TD and AB, and their labeling indices to predict susceptibility of a gland at that stage of development to carcinogenesis. The induction of numerous and varied morphologic lesions in the rat mammary gland appears to be due to the site of origin within the tissue (Russo, Russo, Ireland, Saby 1977; Russo, Saby, Isenberg, Russo 1977; Russo, Wilgus, Russo 1979). The pathologic events resulting from the action of DMBA at the level of the TEB apparently result in adenocarcinomas (Fig. 10). Whereas the interaction of DMBA at the level of the more differentiated portions of the gland, AB and lobules, results in benign lesions as in Fig. 11.

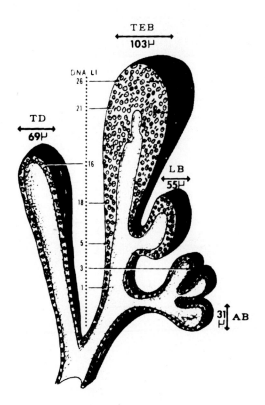

Fig. 9: Schematic representation of the terminal structures of the mammary gland tree of a young virgin rat.
TEB = terminal end bud; TD = terminal duct; LB = lateral
bud; AB = alveolar bud; DNA-LI = DNA labeling index. The
values beneath the two-headed arrows are the average diameter in μ. Reprinted by permission from: (Russo,
Wilgus, Russo 1979).

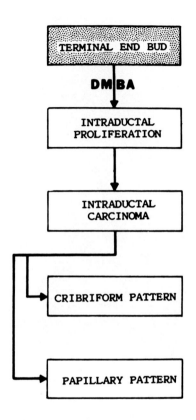

Fig. 10: Pathological events occuring at the level of the terminal end bud after exposure to DMBA. Reprinted by permission from: (Russo, Saby, Isenberg, Russo 1977).

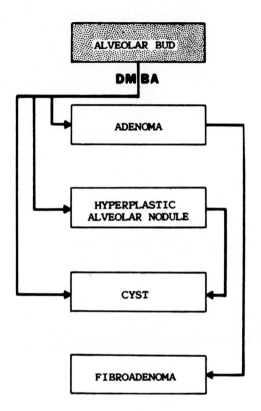

Fig. 11: Pathological events taking place at the level of the alveolar bud after exposure to DMBA. Reprinted by permission from: (Russo, Saby, Isenberg, Russo 1977).

A natural extension of this type of study was to determine if the type or level of dietary fat with which the animal was being fed, both with and without a carcinogenesis-inhibiting antioxidant, influences the development of the virgin mammary gland with respect to the features outlined above and with respect to the age of the animal. Collaborative work done between this laboratory and that of Dr. Russo at the Michigan Cancer Foundation has addressed the specific question of whether or not dietary fat and antioxidants may influence the development of the rat mammary gland. In these studies, weanling rats were placed directly onto their respective diets (5 animals per dietary group) and housed as a single species and sex within a room. The experimental protocol was identical to that of the tumor incidence studies (Part 1 of this article) up to the point of carcinogen treatment, except that at exactly 50 days of age, rather than receiving DMBA, they were sacrificed. Their 4th, 5th, and 6th mammary glands, both left and right sides, were removed, left attached to the skin flap and pinned to cork sheets so that they were flat. They were immediately placed in 10% phosphate-buffered formalin and sent to Dr. Russo's laboratory where characterization of the development of the glands of rats fed the various diets was performed and compared to age-matched chow-fed animals (Russo, Russo 1978b; Russo, Russo 1980). All samples were sent blind and identified only after their characterization had been completed. This information was then related to the sensitivity of the rat mammary glands to carcinogen treatment and concomitant mammary tumor development, i.e. the tumor incidence data.

Dr. Russo has shown that the TEB and TD are the sensitive targets within the mammary gland. The more TEB and TD structure that are present at the time of carcinogen exposure, the higher the incidence of mammary adenocarcinoma. The 50-day-old chow-fed rat possesses a high density of TEB and TD structures which are actively differentiating into AB, and have a high DNA-labeling index (Russo, Russo 1978b; Russo, Wilgus, Russo 1979). The high susceptibility to carcinogenesis that has been demonstrated in young virgin rats appears to be due to the presence of a large proliferative compartment, primarily in the TEB and TD structures. The low susceptibility of parous animals is due to the formation of a large compartment of non-proliferating cells, and those cells which are still pro-

liferating, have a longer G phase than do those of younger and older virgin rats (Russo, Russo 1980).

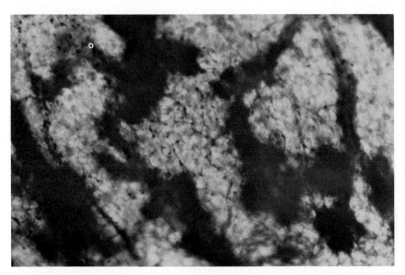

Fig. 12: Wholemount of mammary gland of a 50 day old
female Sprague-Dawley rat consuming a high polyunsaturated
fat diet from weaning (21 days of age). Toluidine blue, x
36.

Animals consuming both the HPF and HSF diets developed glands with numerous TEB and AB with profuse branching
being apparent. Figure 12 shows the appearance of glands
from animals consuming the HPF diet. This figure is a
representative section of a mammary gland whole mount from
these HPF-fed animals and shows the short, profuse
branches characteristic of this group. These glands are
more developed than those of animals consuming the HSF
diet (compare Figure 13). There are some club-shaped TEB,
but the most abundant structures are the early AB, structures that are very susceptible to DMBA carcinogenesis.

Figure 13 is a whole mount mammary gland section from
animals consuming the HSF diet. This shows the short,
wide, and numerous branches which end in either lateral
buds or in club-shaped TEB. Here it is possible to observe the absence of lobules and the more immature appearance of the gland. The development of these glands ap-

pears to be that of a 25-35 day-old chow-fed control animal. The abundance of TEB predicts a high incidence of
tumor development, although with a longer latency.

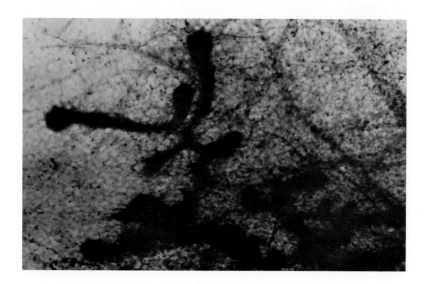

Fig. 13: Wholemount of mammary gland of a 50 day old
female Sprague-Dawley rat consuming a high saturated fat
diet from weaning (21 days of age). Toluidine blue x 36.

Animals consuming the LF diet displayed more heterogeneity in their glandular structure. Some of the glands
of LF-fed animas were well-developed with prominent TEB,
others were more atrophic. Figure 14 is from a LF-fed
animal, demonstrating an atrophic appearance. Results in
this group were routinely split fairly evenly. If animals
spontaneously respond so differently to a low fat diet,
then at least two groups, one with a significant tumor
incidence, and another with a very low mammary tumor incidence, respectively will be found.

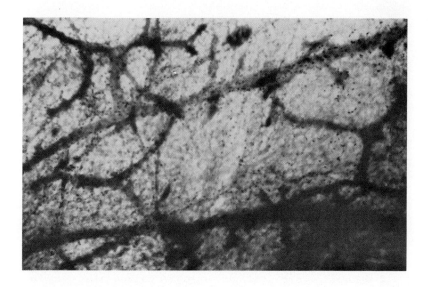

Fig. 14: Wholemount of a mammary gland of a 50 day-old female Sprague-Dawley rat consuming a low-fat diet since weaning (21 days of age). Toluidine blue x 36.

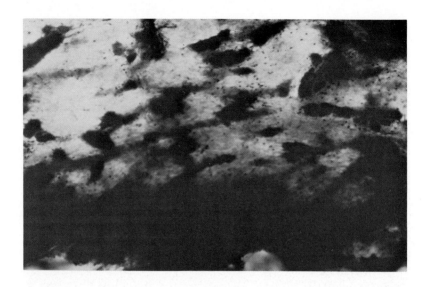

Fig. 15: Wholemount of a mammary gland of a 50 day-old
female Sprague-Dawley rat consuming a polyunsaturated fat
diet + 0.3% BHT since weaning (21 days of age). Toluidine
blue x 36.

     Animals consuming these three diets with 0.3% BHT
supplementation showed quite different appearances from
those of the animals on the corresponding non-supplemented
diets. Those consuming the HPF + BHT diet had glands that
occupied a large area and were composed of long narrow
ducts with occasional lateral branching, and only a moderate number of lateral buds (Figure 15). Ducts distal to
the nipple ended in thin, palely staining TD. Very few
TEB and AB were seen. The development of the mammary
gland in this group of animals corresponded to that of a
100 day-old virgin, in which Russo observed an incidence
of mammary adenocarcinomas in chow-fed animals of 62-66%
(Russo and Russo 1978b). King et al. observed an
incidence of 50-60% in HSF + BHT-fed animals (King,
Bailey, Gibson, Pitha, McCay 1979).

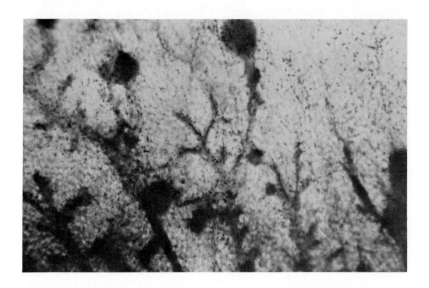

Fig. 16: Wholemount of a mammary gland of a 50 day-old
female Sprague-Dawley rat consuming a high saturated fat
diet supplemented with 0.3% BHT since weaning (21 days of
age). Toluidine blue x 36.

The mammary glands of female rats consuming the HSF +
BHT diet were more heterogeneous. In general, they were
composed of long, thin ducts branching only occasionally,
and with very few lateral buds (Figure 16). Terminal
ducts ended in cystically dilated TEB and TD. The general
appearence overall was atrophic. The presence of cystically dilated TEB, TD, and AB have never been observed in
non-BHT supplemented purified diet-fed animals, or in
chow-fed animals, and suggests that the HSF + BHT diet
could alter the development of these structures, resulting
in their being more refractory to the carcinogen. The
noticeable absence of normal TEB and AB structures could
account for a lower incidence of carcinomas.

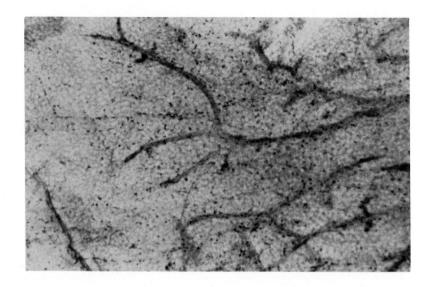

Fig. 17: Wholemount of a mammary gland of a 50 day-old
female Sprague-Dawley rat consuming a low fat diet supplemented with 0.3% BHT since weaning (21 days of age).
Toluidine blue x 36.

        Animals consuming the LF + BHT diet were the most
homogeneous with respect to glandular development. All
the glands were composed of long narrow ducts without
lateral branching or lateral buds (Figure 17). No TEB or
AB were seen. The glands had an atrophic appearance probably due to a lack of progesteronic stimulation. There
was no difference between the glands of animals in pro-
estrous or diestrous (as determined by vaginal smears).
Even the glands of very old virgin rats present more active structures than did these glands. With this structure of the gland being present at the time of DMBA administration, one would expect a very low incidence of tumors
to occur. Indeed, in this group the incidence ranged from
25-35% (King, Bailey, Gibson, Pitha, McCay 1979).

It is apparent that a LF diet, or the addition of 0.3% BHT to the diet, resulted in either more atrophic or more differentiated glands than is normally seen in a 50 day-old chow-fed animal. Both of these features would be predictive of a lower susceptibility to tumor development due to fewer target sites for interaction of the etiologic agent. The HPF and HSF diet-fed animals on the other hand have glands which are considerably more undifferentiated (many TEB and AB) at 50 days of age, allowing for more potential target sites and a resulting higher tumor incidence following exposure to a carcinogenic substance. Other factors altering susceptibility to carcinogens are no doubt operative, but these diet-dependent developmental differences must account for at least part of the large differences in mammary tumor incidence in female rats treated with the same amount of carcinogen at the same chronological age.

ACKNOWLEDGEMENTS

We wish to thank Ms. Gemma Brueggemann, Ms. Jo Johnson, Mr. Tim Wilkins and Mr. Larry Leemaster for their excellent technical assistance. The authors wish to thank Ms. Sherie Loman, Kay Wallace and Lisa Gropf for help in the typing and preparation of this manuscript. This work supported in part by NIH Grants # ES01789 to M. King and # CA23529 to I. Russo.

REFERENCES

Aaes-Jorgensen E (1961). Essential Fatty Acids. Physiol Rev 41:1.

Astwood EB, Geschickter CF, Rausch EO (1937). Development of the Mammary Gland of the Rat. Am J Anatomy 61:373.

Benson T, Lev M Grand CG (1956). Enhancement of Mammary Fibroadenomas in the Female Rat by a High Fat Diet. Cancer   Res 16:135.

Bieri JG, Briggs GM, Pollard CJ, Spivey-Fox MR (1960). Normal Growth and Development of Female Chickens without Dietary Vitamin E or Other Antioxidants. J Nutr 70:47.

Boice JD, Monson RR (1977). Breast Cancer in Women After Repeated Fluoroscopic Examinations of the Chest. J Natl Cancer Inst 59:823.

Carroll KK (1975). Experimental Evidence of Dietary Factors and Hormone-Dependent Cancers. Cancer Res 35: 3374.

Carroll KK, Gammal EB, Plunkett ER (1968). Dietary Fat and Mammary Cancer. Canad Med Assn J 98:590.

Chan PC, Dao TL (1981). Enhancement of Mammary Carcinogenesis by a High-Fat Fed Diet in Fischer, Long-Evans, and Sprague-Dawley Rats. Cancer Res 41:164.

Craig TJ, Comstock SW, Geisen RB (1974). Epidemiologic Comparison of Breast Cancer Patients with Early and Late Onset of Malignancy and General Population Controls. J Natl Cancer Inst 53:1577.

Dam H (1957). Influence of Antioxidants and Redox Substances on Signs of Vitamin E Deficiency. Pharmacol Rev 9:1.

Dao TL (1964). Carcinogenesis of Mammary Gland in Rat. Progr Exp Tumor Res 5:157.

Draper HH, Csallany AS (1958). Action of N,N'-diphenyl-p-phenylenediamine in Tocopherol Deficiency Diseases. Proc Soc Expt'l Biol Med 99:739.

Engel RW, Copeland DH (1951). Influence of Diet on the Relative Incidence of Eye, Mammary, Ear-duct, and Liver Tumors in Rats Fed 2-Acetylaminofluorene. Cancer Res 11:180.

Gammal EB, Carroll KK, Plunkett ER (1967). Effect of Dietary Fat on Mammary Carcinogenesis by 7,12-dimethylbenz(α)anthracene in Rats. Cancer Res 27:17371

Horwitt MK (1970). "Tocopherol and Polyunsaturated Fatty Acid Relationships" In Shimazono N, Takagi Y (eds): "International Symposium on Vitamin E," Tokyo: Kyoritsu Chuppan Co. Ltd., pp. 45.

Huggins C, Grand LC, Brillantes FP (1959). Critical Significance of Breast Structure in the Induction of Mammary Cancer in the Rat. Proc Natl Acad Sci 45:1294.

Huggins C, Grand LC, Brillantes FP (1967). Mammary Cancer Induced by a Single Feeding of Polynuclear Hydrocarbons and its Suppression. Nature 189:204.

Juret P, Couette JE, Mandard AM, Carre A, Delozier T, Brune D, Vernhes J (1976). Age and Menarche as a Prognostic Factor in Human Breast Cancer. Eur J Cancer 12:701.

King MM, Bailey DM, Gibson DD, Pitha JV, McCay PB (1979). The Incidence and Growth of Mammary Tumors Induced by 7,12-dimethylbenz(α)anthracene as related to the Dietary Content of Fat and Antioxidant. J Natl Cancer Inst 63:657.

King MM, McCay PB (1981). Studies on Liver Microsomes of Female Rats Fed Purified Diets Varying in Fat Content With and Without Propyl Gallate. Food Cosmet Toxicol 19:13.

Kinoshita N, Gelboin HV (1972). The Role of Aryl Hydrocarbon Hydroxylase in 7,12-Dimethylbenz(α)anthracene Skin Tumorigenesis: On the Mechanism of 7,8-Benzoflavone Inhibition of Tumorigenesis. Cancer Res 32:1329.

McGregor DH, Land CE, Choi K, Tokjoka S, Lui PI, Wakabayashie T, Beebe GW (1977). Breast Cancer Incidence Among Atomic Bomb Survivors, Hiroshima & Nagasaki. J Natl Cancer Inst 59:799.

MacMahon B, Cole P, Brown J (1973). Etiology of Human Breast Cancer: A Review. J Natl Cancer Inst 50:21.

MacMahon B, Cole P, Lin M, Lowe CR, Mirra AP, Ravinihar B, Salber EJ, Valaoras VG, Yvasa S (1970). Age at First Birth and Breast Cancer Risk. Bull W H O 34:209.

Moon RC (1969). Relationship Between Previous Reproductive History and Chemically Induced Mammary Cancer in Rats. Int J Cancer 4:312.

Mohrhauer H, Holman RT (1963). The Effect of Dose Level of Essential Fatty Acids upon Fatty Composition of the Liver. J Lipid Res 4:151.

Murad T, von Haam E (1972). Studies of Mammary Carcinoma Induced by 7,12-dimethylbenz(α)anthracene Administration. Cancer Res 32:1404.

Norkin SA (1966). Lipid Nature of Ceroid in Experimental Nutritional Cirrhosis. Arch Path 82:259.

Pappenheimer AM, Goetsch M (1931). A Cerebellar Disorder in Chicks Apparently of Nutritional Origin. J Expt'l Med 53:11.

Richards J, Nandi S (1978). Primary Culture of Rat Mammary Epithelial Cells. II Cytotoxic Effect and Metabolism of 7,12-Dimethylbanz(α)anthracene and N-Nitroso-N-Methylurea. J Nat'l Cancer Inst 61:773.

Russo J, Russo IH, Ireland M, Saby J (1977). Increased Resistance of Multiparous Rat Mammary Gland to Neoplastic Transformation by 7,12-dimethylbenz(α)anthracene. Proc Am Assoc Cancer Res 18:38.

Russo J, Saby J, Isenberg WM, Russo IH (1977). Pathogenesis of Mammary Carcinomas Induced in Rats by 7,12-dimethylbenz(α)anthracene. J Natl Cancer Inst 59:435.

Russo IH, Russo J (1978a). Developmental Stage of the Rat Mammary Gland as Determinant of Its Susceptibility to 7,12-dimethylbenz(α)anthracene. J Natl Cancer Inst 61:1439.

Russo J, Russo IH (1978b). DNA Labeling Index and Structure of the Rat Mammary Gland as Determinants of Its Susceptibility to Carcinogenesis. J Natl Cancer Inst 61:1451.

Russo J, Russo IH (1980). Influence of Differentiation and Cell Kinetics on the Susceptibility of the Rat Mammary Gland to Carcinogenesis. Cancer Res 40:2677.

Russo J, Wilgus G, Russo IH (1979). Susceptibility of the Mammary Gland to Carcinogenesis. I. Differentiation of the Mammary Gland as Determinant of Tumor Incidence and Type of Lesion. Am J Pathol 96:721.

Schwarz K (1952). Sulfer-containing Amino Acids and Vitamin E in Dietary Liver Necrosis. Fed Proc 11:455.

Silverstone H, Tannenbaum A (1950). The Effect of the Proportion of Dietary Fat on the Rate of Formation of Mammary Carcinoma in Mice. Cancer Res 10:448.

Slaga TJ, Klein-Syanto AJP, Triplett LL, Yotti LP, Trosko JE (1981). Skin Tumor-Promoting Activity of Benzoyl Peroxide, a Widely Used Free Radical-Generating Compound. Science 213:1023.

Tannenbaum A (1945). The Dependence of Tumor Formation on the Composition of the Calorie-Restricted Diet as well as on the Degree of Restriction. Cancer Res 5:616.

Vasington FD, Reichard SM, Nason A (1960). Biochemistry of Vitamin E. Vit and Horm 18:43.

Wattenberg LW (1978). Inhibition of Chemical Carcinogenesis. J Nat'l Cancer Inst 60:11.

Witting LA (1969). The Oxidation of α-Tocopherol during the Autoxidation of Ethyl Oleate, Linoleate, Linolenate, and Arachidonate. Arch Biochem Biophys 129:142.

Witting LA (1979). Vitamin E-Polyunsaturated Lipid Relationship in diet and Tissues. Amer J Clin Nutr 27:952.

Wynder EL (1976). Nutrition and Cancer. Fed Proc 35:1309.

RETINOIDS AND CANCER

Diet, Nutrition, and Cancer:
From Basic Research to Policy Implications, pages 93–94
© *1983 Alan R. Liss, Inc., 150 Fifth Avenue, New York, NY 10011*

RETINOIDS AND CANCER
Chairman's Introduction

George Wolf, D.Phil.

Department of Nutrition and Food Science
Massachusetts Institute of Technology
Cambridge, MA 02139

Gradually, looking over the evidence, I have come to
the conclusion that there are at least two separate biochemical functions of vitamin A, outside of the process of
vision; one is via the nucleus and one is extranuclear,
possibly through action on the cell surface. I wish I
could use Occam's razor and thereby minimize the number of
hypotheses by stating that the two known active forms of
vitamin A, retinol and retinoic acid, each controls one of
the two functions. Alas, this cannot be done. There is
no compelling evidence that retinol or retinoic acid acts
preferentially by one or the other mechanism.

Vitamin A is necessary for normal differentiation of
epithelia. In cell culture systems, vitamin A can direct
differentiation of keratocytes by controlling keratin mRNA
transcription or stability or processing. Differentiation
of embryonal carcinoma cells into parietal endoderm can be
induced by retinoic acid, also with induction of mRNA for
specific endodermal proteins. Thus, at least in these two
systems, there is a clear effect of the vitamin on the cell
nucleus.

On the other hand, vitamin A can suppress the effects
of tumor promoters, at the same time as inducing changes
in cell-surface glycoproteins. These have been well characterized in some cases, such as in that of the cell-surface
glycoprotein fibronectin. This glycoprotein is necessary
for cell adhesion to substratum, and is lost as a result
of promoter treatment. Retinoids can prevent this loss.
In our laboratory, we have used enucleated cells which also

lose fibronectin when treated with promoter. Even in these cells, lacking a nucleus, retinoids can counteract the promoter effect on fibronectin. Thus, without a doubt, in some functions, vitamin A can act in an extranuclear way, most probably by a cell-surface function.

This workshop panel has been selected to address these different functions of the retinoids: the nuclear function and differentiation, and the glycoprotein function and tumor promotion. Finally, the application of this knowledge to the human situation in terms of the epidemiology of cancer in relation to dietary vitamin A will be discussed.

Diet, Nutrition, and Cancer:
From Basic Research to Policy Implications, pages 95–109
© *1983 Alan R. Liss, Inc., 150 Fifth Avenue, New York, NY 10011*

RETINOIDS AND TUMOR PROMOTION

Stuart H. Yuspa, M.D.

Chief, Laboratory of Cellular Carcinogenesis
and Tumor Promotion, National Cancer Institute
Bethesda, MD 20205

During the last decade considerable progress has occurred in the area of experimental chemical carcinogenesis. Of
particular significance has been the development of animal
models for most major target sites of carcinogenesis in man.
Cancer development in these animal models strongly parallels
the pathogenesis of cancer in the analogous human tissue and
and is likely to be mechanistically similar (Yuspa and Harris,
1982). These models have fulfilled an indispensible pre-
requisite for the development of cancer prevention protocols.

The availability of appropriate animal models has greatly
facilitated the search for agents which could inhibit chemical
carcinogenesis. Inhibitors are important for potential chemoprevention of human cancer but also serve as probes to determine factors which are mechanistically relevant in cancer
development. Vitamin A first showed evidence of having a protective effect on carcinogenesis in several stratified squamous epithelia (Bollag, 1972; Chu and Malmgren, 1965; Davies,
1967). These initial observations have now been extended to
include other model systems and a number of natural and
synthetic retinoids (Sporn and Newton, 1981). Table 1 indicates animal model systems where retinoids have reproducibly
exerted an inhibitory action on carcinogenesis. Kinetic
studies on the role of retinoids in these models have indicated that their inhibitory effects are largely in the post
initiation or post carcinogen exposure portion of the carcinogenesis protocol (McCormick et al., 1980, 1981; Moon et al.,
1977; Nettesheim et al., 1976; Nettesheim and Williams,
1976; Saffiotti et al., 1967; Sporn et al., 1977; Verma and
Boutwell, 1977). Retinoids are effective by systemic or

Table 1. Retinoid Influence on the Post Initiation

Phase of Carcinogenesis

Inhibition

Mouse skin
Rat mammary gland
Rat bladder
Rat lung (hamster lung)

No effect or enhancement

Hamster trachea
Rat colon
Mouse mammary gland
Mouse skin

topical exposures in these models. It should be noted that
those tissues in which retinoids are pharmacologically effective as tumor inhibitors (Table 1) are also targets for the
physiological influences of retinoids on growth and differentiation. Animal studies have also indicated that under certain treatment conditions, retinoids may have no effect or
can enhance carcinogenesis. These paradoxical results have
sometimes been observed in the same target tissue in which
inhibitory activity has been demonstrated (Table 1 and
Hennings et al., 1982; Schroder and Black, 1980; Silverman
et al., 1981; Stinson et al., 1981; Welsch et al., 1981) and
have complicated approaches to understand the mechanism of
retinoid action. Such ambiguities have prompted caution in
the use of retinoids for clinical purposes.

Of all the model systems currently used to study retinoids and carcinogenesis, mouse skin is probably the best
understood and most adaptable for research. This model can
be divided into operationally and mechanistically distinct
stages, initiation and promotion (Yuspa, 1981-1982). Results
from several laboratories concerning the modifying role of
retinoids in this model are summarized in Table 2. Retinoids
are potent inhibitors of phorbol ester promotion (Bollag,
1972; Verma and Boutwell, 1977) but do not influence the
initiation phase of skin carcinogenesis (Verma et al., 1979;
Verma et al., 1980). When promotion is subdivided into early
and late stages, dependent on the ability of specific chemical agents to complete the process (Slaga et al., 1980a),

Table 2.   Retinoids and Mouse Skin Tumorigenesis

1.   Phorbol ester mediated tumor promotion is inhibited by
     retinoids.
2.   Inhibition is most effective in later stages of promotion.
3.   Retinoids must be applied within a few hours of promoter
     exposure.
4.   Phorbol ester receptor binding is not altered.
5.   Phorbol ester induced ornithine decarboxylase (ODC)
     activity and putrescine accumulation are completely
     inhibited.
6.   Phorbol ester induced hyperplasia is not affected.
7.   When exposed to retinoids, existing skin tumors may
     regress without a change in cell proliferation rate.
8.   Retinoids do not inhibit (but may enhance) complete
     carcinogenesis by polycyclic aromatic hydrocarbons.
9.   Under appropriate exposure conditions, retinoids are
     tumor promoters.

retinoids are effective only in the later stage (Slaga et al.,
1980b).   There is a strict time dependence with regard to
applications of retinoids and promoters.   Retinoid exposure
must occur shortly prior to or after phorbol esters to be
effective in blocking promotion (Verma et al., 1978).   This
time dependence does not seem to relate to an effect of retinoids on phorbol ester binding to its receptor (Solanki
et al., 1981).   Retinoids are potent inhibitors of phorbol
ester induced ornithine decarboxylase (ODC) activity and
there is a strong association for a series of synthetic retinoids to inhibit both ODC and tumor promotion (Verma and
Boutwell, 1977; Verma et al., 1978).   However retinoids do
not influence the hyperplastic response to phorbol esters
(Verma, 1981).   While retinoids are extremely effective at
preventing tumor formation in skin, they are also potent at
causing regression of existing tumors (Bollag, 1972, 1975).
The mechanism of this effect is obscure since retinoids do not
significantly alter the proliferation rate of existing tumors
(Frigg and Torhorst, 1977).   There appears to be a specific
effect on the most differentiated cells in the tumor mass
since both the granular cell layer and stratum corneum are
markedly diminished in retinoid treated tumors (Frigg and
Torhorst, 1977).   Epithelial necrosis and stromal enlarge-
ment are also observed (Frigg and Torhorst, 1977; Mori and
Kabayashi, 1981).   It is particularly noteworthy that retinoids are ineffective and in fact may enhance tumorigenesis

(both benign and malignant tumors) induced by repeated application of polycyclic aromatic hydrocarbons (Verma et al., 1982). This implies a specific effect on the promoting action of phorbol esters. This specific mechanism of action is further emphasized by the finding that retinoids alone, if given repeatedly, can act as tumor promoters in the same concentrations which when given with phorbol esters are inhibitory to tumor promotion (Hennings et al., 1982).

In order to understand the function of retinoids in tumor promotion, scrutiny of the biological characteristics of skin tumor promotion is required. Table 3 presents some of these

Table 3: Characteristics of Mouse Skin Tumor Promotion

1. Tumors are produced only in initiated skin.
2. Promoters must be applied repeatedly and at frequent intervals.
3. Benigh tumors (papillomas) are the major neoplasms.
4. Malignant tumors are rare, arise from papillomas, occur late and develop independent of continued promoter exposure.
5. Tumors are monoclonal
6. Promoter stimulated biochemical changes occur in many cells, not just initiated cells.
7. Cell selection or tissue sensitization leads to enhanced responses with multiple promoter applications.

characteristics. Promotion is effective only in previously initiated skin and promoters must be applied repeatedly. Thus individual promoter exposures are reversible. Protocols in mouse skin using promoting agents are effective at producing premalignant lesions (papillomas) and are inefficient at producing malignant tumors although carcinomas ultimately arise from some papillomas even long after promotion has been terminated. The tumors which develop in skin carcinogenesis are monoclonal presumeably arising from single initiated cells (Iannaccone et al., 1978). Promoters induce biochemical changes in many or all epidermal cells not just initiated cells. Repeated promoter exposure sensitizes the tissue for certain responses to a subsequent exposure such as stimulation of DNA synthesis (Raick et al., 1972), stimulation of ODC induction (O'Brien, 1976) and elevation of cyclic guanosine monophosphate levels (Garte and Belman, 1978). This suggests a greater proportion of sensitive cells populate the epidermis during promotion. The monoclonal origin of tumors, the suggestion of tissue remodeling with repetitive promoter exposure and the requirement for repeated promoting stimuli prior to the development of tumors strongly suggest that cell selection is involved in promotion. It is within this framework that we must consider the role of retinoids.

Our laboratory has utilized cultured mouse epidermal cells to facilitate studies on the mechanisms of initiation and promotion of carcinogenesis. During the development and application of this model we have emphasized the close biological and biochemical parallels of skin in vivo and epidermal cells in culture (Yuspa et al., 1980b). A major advance in epidermal cell culture came with the discovery that extracellular ionic calcium is a key regulator of epi-

dermal growth and differentiation (Hennings et al., 1980). In medium with reduced calcium concentrations (0.02-0.09 mM), epidermal basal cells are selectively cultivated. These cells have morphological, cell kinetic and marker protein characteristics of basal cells and grow as a monolayer with a high proliferation rate. When the calcium concentration of culture medium is elevated to levels found in most commercial preparations (1.2-1.4 mM), proliferation ceases and terminal differentiation rapidly ensues with squamous differentiation and sloughing of cells occurring by 72-96 hours. This simple physiological manipulation has been useful in approaching questions regarding initiation and promotion.

In the last several years studies utilizing this model have allowed us to develop a working hypothesis on the biological basis of initiation and promotion in mouse skin. These hypotheses are based on our current understanding of the regulation of growth and differentiation of normal epidermis. In vivo, only a small number of epidermal basal cells proliferate at a particular time and those which leave the basement membrane are obligated to terminally differentiate. In epidermal tumors (both papillomas and carcinomas), the proliferating population increases 10 fold and proliferating cells are observed away from the basement membrane area (Burns et al., 1976). In papillomas other characteristics of epidermal differentiation are maintained (Raick, 1973). This suggests that during the process of carcinogenesis, an alteration occurs in initiated cells (the clonal expansion of which we presume forms papillomas) that is expressed as

the ability to proliferate under conditions where normal
cells cannot or where normal cells are obligated to differentiate. The responses of cultured basal cells to increases
in extracellular calcium resemble the events associated with
the commitment to differentiate and to migrate away from the
basement membrane in vivo. It might be expected, in analogy
with in vivo data, that carcinogens could alter the basal
cell response to calcium induced terminal differentiation.

A variety of studies to probe this possibility have been
performed in our laboratory. Basal cells exposed to carcinogens in vitro and subsequently induced to differentiate by
calcium formed foci which resisted terminal differentiation
(Kulesz-Martin et al., 1980). Colony number was proportional
to carcinogen dose. Cells obtained from these colonies demonstrated epithelial morphology and expressed differentiative
functions but failed to cease proliferation when signaled to
differentiate. Such cell lines derived from these assays
were not tumorigenic when initially tested, but on prolonged
subculture the majority yielded tumorigenic cell lines. All
lines have a unimodal DNA content suggesting they are clonal
in origin. Similar foci were derived from cell cultures of
mouse skin initiated in vivo by exposure of mice to 7,12-
dimethylbenz[a]anthracene and subsequent culture of epidermis
in 0.02 mM calcium medium for several weeks followed by
selection in 1.2 mM calcium. In these experiments control
skin did not yield colonies (Yuspa and Morgan, 1981). These
results suggest that initiation of carcinogenesis results in
the ability of initiated cells to resist the signal to cease
proliferation in association with terminal differentiation.
In normal skin such a trait alone could not result in a tumor
due to the strong regulatory influences of surrounding normal
cells, since normal epidermal proliferation and maturation
are confined to unit structures regulated by adjacent units
(Potten 1974, Potten and Allen 1975). Thus deviant behavior
of an individual cell would be restricted to a single unit
and regulated by the division and maturation rate of surrounding units. If initiation is an infrequent event, change
in proliferative capacity in only a small number of units
would be nearly impossible to detect experimentally in vivo
in the absence of tumor promotion but could be expressed
during the calcium selection exerted by our in vitro assay.

Recent studies in culture have also indicated a mechanism
whereby tumor promoters could act to select for initiated
cells and cause their clonal expansion. Basal cell cultures,

exposed to the potent tumor promoter 12-0-tetradecanoylphor-bol-13-acetate (TPA) and maintained in 0.07 mM Ca^{++}, rapidly undergo a morphological change in which a portion of the cell population becomes rounded and eventually detaches from the monolayer. Detaching cells are cornified and the process is associated with a substantial increase in epidermal trans-glutaminase activity (Yuspa et al., 1980a). This effect does not appear to be the result of cytotoxicity but rather a programmed response to TPA in which terminal differentiation is induced in a subclass of basal cells. Other basal cells in the same culture look relatively unaffected by TPA. Thus within the basal cell population, variability in pharmaco-logical responsiveness is easily documented.

When basal cells resistant to the differentiation in-ducing effects of TPA were washed free of cornified cells and studied further, it was found that they were stimulated to proliferate by TPA (Yuspa et al., 1982a). Furthermore these cells were transiently resistant to the differentiation inducing effects of either TPA or 1.2 mM Ca^{++}. If TPA treated cells were allowed to grow for 10 days in 0.02 mM Ca^{++} medium with no further treatment, pharmacological heterogeneity was again restored. Similar studies on a limited number of initi-ated cell lines have indicated that these lines are resistant to the differentiation inducing effects of TPA but responsive to the proliferative influences.

These studies demonstrate the ability of phorbol esters to produce a balanced and programmed heterogeneous response in mouse epidermis with regard to differentiation and proli-feration. Such responses would result in a significant growth advantage to the growth-stimulated population, including initiated cells, at the same time space was provided for cell proliferation along the basement membrane because of the loss of some basal cells by induced differentiation and migration out of the basal layer. In this way initiated cells would clonally expand and repeated selection pressure would yield a benign tumor which is the major lesion in two stage carcino-genesis. Our model requires that a subsequent change in a papilloma cell is necessary for carcinoma development. These concepts previously presented in more detail (Yuspa et al., 1981a; Yuspa et al., 1982a) indicate a critical role of epidermal differentiation in the processes of initiation and promotion of carcinogenesis.

Retinoids are logical agents to alter skin carcinogenesis by virtue of their modifying role in squamous differentiation. The data in Table 2 indicate that two functions of retinoids must be considered in their antineoplastic activity, the ability to antagonize the effects of phorbol esters and the ability to cause tumor regression, this latter effect suggesting a direct action on initiated cells. We have used our cell culture system to study these functions. In one set of experiments (Lichti et al., 1981a) we have shown that basal cells, cultured in low calcium medium, are particularly responsive to the induction of ODC activity by TPA and that inducibility is lost shortly after these cells are committed to differentiate. Additional studies in culture have shown that retinoids are relatively specific for inhibiting ODC activity induced by TPA. Ornithine decarboxylase activity induced by ultraviolet light is much less sensitive to retinoid inhibition (Lichti et al., 1981b). Other inhibitors of ODC (protease inhibitors, local anesthetics) are equally potent for both TPA and ultraviolet light induced activity. These results suggest a specific antagonism of retinoids for certain effects of phorbol esters and also imply that basal cells are the responsive target cells for both TPA and retinoids. We have also reported that retinoids have little effect on TPA stimulated DNA synthesis in cultured epidermal cells until concentrations of $>10^{-5}$M are used (Yuspa et al., 1981). Thus retinoids dissociate ODC activity from proliferation much the same way, but in reverse, as steroid hormones, another group of potent inhibitors of skin tumor promotion (Lichti et al., 1977).

While both ODC and DNA synthesis are involved in proliferative functions in skin, differentiative functions are critical to promotion. In our working hypothesis, the induction of differentiation by phorbol esters is essential to produce the loss of normal cells required for clonal expansion of initiated cells. Induction of epidermal differentiation has been documented in our culture model by studying the increase in the activity of the differentiation enzyme, epidermal transglutaminase, in basal cells exposed to phorbol esters (Yuspa et al., 1980). Transglutaminase is a calcium dependent cytosolic enzyme which catalyzes the formation of the ε(γ-glutamyl-lysine) dipeptide bond in the cross linked cornified envelope in epidermal cells. The activity of this enzyme is low in cultured basal cells but increases with calcium induced differentiation (Hennings et al., 1981). Basal cell cultures exposed to phorbol esters show a significant increase in this enzyme activity and a marked increase in cornified cells which are lost from the culture dish (Yuspa et al., 1982a). As cornified cells are removed from the attached population of basal cells, transglutaminase activity returns to basal levels (Yuspa et al., 1980a). We have studied the effect of retinoids on this enzyme and on the differentiation inducing activity of phorbol esters. Surprisingly, retinoic acid is a potent inducer of transglutaminase. Induction is dose and time dependent, but unlike the induction by phorbol ester, activity remains high throughout the course of exposure (Table 4) (Yuspa et al., 1982b). Combined exposure to phorbol ester and retinoic acid are not additive (Table 4). When cells are exposed to both TPA and retinoic acid, activity of transglutaminase increases but remains elevated, unlike the transient increase seen with TPA alone (Table 4). Transglutaminase activity induced by either retinoic acid or TPA appears to be due to the same enzyme since many characteristics are identical including substrate Km (Yuspa et al., 1982b).

This increase in transglutaminase activity induced by retinoic acid was particularly puzzling since we had previously shown that similar concentrations of the retinoid blocked epidermal differentiation by calcium (Yuspa et al., 1981b). When cornification was studied in retinoid treated basal cells induced to differentiate by calcium, we found a dramatic reduction in cornified cells (Yuspa et al., 1982b). Furthermore, the formation of the isodipeptide bond was strongly inhibited (Yuspa et al., 1982b). Thus retinoids have a novel mechanism of altering epidermal differentiation whereby they increase transglutaminase activity but block cornification. This suggested that retinoids could influence cell loss in phorbol ester treated epidermal cells since the mechanism of loss was related to accelerated cornification. Epidermal cells induced to differentiate by calcium were also exposed to both retinoic acid and TPA or TPA alone, and DNA or protein per dish was measured over time. TPA alone caused a dramatic loss of both DNA and protein as differentiating cells sloughed from the culture dish. Retinoic acid prevented this cell loss as indicated by the stability of DNA or protein per dish in cells receiving both TPA and retinoic acid (Table 5). Thus it appears that retinoids, by inhibiting the cornification process, can interfere with an essential biological function of phorbol ester tumor promoters, the induction of terminal differentiation.

Table 4. Induction of Epidermal Transglutaminase by 12-0-tetradecanoylphorbol-13-acetate (TPA) and Retinoic Acid (RA)

Experiment	Epidermal Transglutaminase (CPM/mg Protein/10 min x 10^{-3})[a]						

1. Timecourse (Hrs)

	0	2	4	6	8	12	24
TPA (1.7 x 10^{-7}M)	1.2	1.2	1.2	1.5	3.0	4.4	2.4
RA (10^{-6}M)	1.3	1.2	-	1.4	2.2	3.0	4.5

2. Dose-Response (M)

	0	10^{-9}	10^{-8}	10^{-7}	10^{-6}	10^{-5}
TPA (x 1.6)	2.6	2.6	3.5	7.2	3.6	-
RA (x 1)	3.8	5.0	6.2	6.2	15.2	15.0

3. Combined Treatment Timecourse (Hrs)[b]

	0	4	8	14	24	32
TPA (1.6 x 10^{-7}M)	1.7	2.0	3.5	5.6	3.4	2.8
RA (10^{-6}M) + TPA (1.6 x 10^{-7}M)	4.2	3.7	4.8	4.8	4.4	4.8

a. Determined as the Ca^{++} dependent incorporation of ^{3}H-putrescine into casein in cell lysates as described in Yuspa et al., 1980a. All experiments were conducted in 0.07 mM Ca^{++} medium on primary cultures of Balb/c newborn mouse epidermal cells.

b. RA exposure was for 24 hours prior to TPA as well as during TPA exposure. Zero time refers to the beginning of treatment with TPA. In RA pretreated cells transglutaminase activity is already elevated by zero time.

TABLE 5. Protective Effect of Retinoic Acid Against Cell
Loss Induced by Tumor Promoters[a]

Treatment Group	Time (Hrs)					
	0	12	24	48	72	96
	μg protein/dish					
TPA (1.7 x 10^{-7}M)	283	265	189	83	58	104
RA (10^{-6}M) + TPA (1.7 x 10^{-7}M)	377	383	344	326	248	324

a. Basal cells (0.07 mM Ca^{++} medium) were pretreated with
10^{-6}M retinoic acid or 0.1% DMSO (solvent) for 24 hours and
then exposed to TPA in medium containing 1.2 mM Ca^{++} to
induce differentiation. Exposure to TPA or TPA + RA was for
24 hours after which fresh medium (1.2 mM Ca^{++}) containing
either RA or DMSO was applied every 24 hours. Duplicate
samples were removed at the indicated times and total protein
per dish analyzed as previously described (Lichti et al.,
1981b). Variability among duplicates was < $\pm$ 10%. Similar
results were obtained when DNA per dish was measured.

These studies demonstrate that retinoids have several
potential sites of action as inhibitors of skin carcinogenesis. Mechanistic studies must be conducted within a
framework of understanding of the relevant biology of tumor
promotion. The epidermal cell culture model system is particularly useful to explore this biology in a valid and relevant
manner. Our studies suggest a role of retinoids in modulating
the differentiation effects of tumor promoters. Currently
we are exploring the biochemistry of this process. Other
studies in our laboratory are focusing on specific retinoid
effects on initiated cell lines. In this way we hope to
understand how retinoids cause regression of tumors.

Bollag, W (1972). Prophylaxis of chemically induced benign
and malignant epithelial tumors by vitamin A acid (retinoic
acid). Europ J Cancer 8: 689.
Bollag, W (1975) Prophylaxis of chemically induced epithelial
tumors with an aromatic retinoic acid analog (Ro 10-9359).
Europ J Cancer 11: 721.

Burns, F J, Vanderlaan, M, Sivak, A, Albert, R A (1976).
Regression kinetics of mouse skin papillomas. Cancer Res
36: 1422.

Chu, E W, Malmgren, R A (1965). An inhibitory effect of
vitamin A on the induction of tumors of forestomach and
cervix in the syrian hamster by carcinogenic polycyclic
hydrocarbons. Cancer Res 25: 884.

Davies, R E (1967). Effect of vitamin A on 7,12-dimethyl-
benz(a)anthracene-induced papillomas in rhino mouse skin.
Cancer Res 27: 237.

Frigg, M, Tohorst, J (1977). Autoradiographic and histopatho-
logic studies on the mode of action of an aromatic retinoid
(Ro 10-9359) on chemically induced epithelial tumors in
Swiss mice. J Natl Cancer Inst 58: 1365.

Garte, S J, Belman, S (1978). Effects of multiple phorbol
myristate acetate treatments on cyclic nucleotide levels in
mouse epidermis. Biochem Biophys Res Commun 84: 489.

Hennings, H, Steinert, P, Buxman, M M (1981) Calcium induction
of transglutaminase and the formation of ε(γ-glutamyl)-
lysine crosslinks in cultured mouse epidermal cells.
Biochem Biophys Res Commun 102: 739.

Hennings, H, Michael, D, Cheng, C, Steinert, P, Holbrook, K,
Yuspa, S (1980). Calcium regulation of growth and differentiation of mouse epidermal cells in culture. Cell 19: 245.

Hennings, H, Wenk, M, Donahoe, R (1982). Retinoic acid
promotion of papilloma formation in mouse skin. Cancer Lett
16: 1-5.

Iannaccone, P M, Gardner, R L, Harris, H (1978). The cellular
origin of chemically induced tumors. J Cell Sci 29: 249.

Kulesz-Martin, M, Koehler, B, Hennings, H, Yuspa, S H (1980).
Quantitative assay for carcinogen altered differentiation
in mouse epidermal cells. Carcinogenesis 1: 995.

Lichti, U, Patterson, E, Hennings, H, Yuspa, S H (1981a).
The tumor promoter 12-0-tetradecanoylphorbol-13-acetate
induced ornithine decarboxylase in proliferating basal cells
but not in differentiating cells from mouse epidermis.
J Cell Physiol 107: 261.

Lichti, U, Patterson, E, Hennings, H, Yuspa, S H (1981b).
Differential retinoic acid inhibition of ornithine decarboxylase induction by 12-0-tetradecanoylphorbol-13-acetate
and by germacidal ultraviolet light. Cancer Res 41: 49.

Lichti, U, Slaga, T J, Ben, T, Patterson, E, Hennings, H,
Yuspa, S H (1977). Dissociation of tumor promoter-stimu-
lated ornithine decarboxylase activity and DNA synthesis
in mouse epidermis in vivo and in vitro by fluocinolone
acetonide, a tumor promotion inhibitor. Proc Natl Acad
Sci USA 74: 3908.

McCormick, D, Burns, F, Albert, R (1980). Inhibition of rat mammary carcinogenesis by short dietary exposure to retinyl acetate. Cancer Res 40: 1140.

McCormick, D, Burns, F, Albert, R (1981). Inhibition of benzo-[a]pyrene-induced mammary carcinogenesis by retinyl acetate. J Natl Cancer Inst 66: 559.

Moon, R, Grubbs, C (1977). Retinyl acetate inhibits mammary carcinogenesis induced by N-methyl-N-nitrosourea. Nature 267: 620.

Mori, M, Kabayashi, K (1981). Histochemical studies on the effect of antitumor retinoid (RO 10-9359) on chemically induced epithelial tumors of the mouse skin. Cell Mol Biol 27: 27.

Nettesheim, P, Cone, M, Snyder, C (1976). The influence of retinyl acetate on the postinitiation phase of preneoplastic lung nodules in rats. Cancer Res 36: 996.

Nettesheim, P, Williams, M (1976). The influence of vitamin A on the susceptibility of the rat lung to 3-methylchol-anthrene. Int J Cancer 17: 351.

O'Brien, T G (1976). The induction of ornithine decarboxy-lase as an early, possibly obligatory, event in mouse skin carcinogenesis. Cancer Res 36: 2644.

Potten, C S (1974). The epidermal proliferative unit: the possible role of the central basal cell. Cell Tissue Kinet 7: 77.

Potten, C S, Allen, T D (1975). Control of epidermal prolife-rative units. Differentiat 3: 161.

Raick, A N (1973). Late ultrastructural changes induced by 12-0-tetradecanoylphorbol-13-acetate and their reversal. Cancer Res 33: 1096.

Raick, A N, Thumm, K, Chivers, B R (1972). Early effects of 12-0-tetradecanoylphorbol-13-acetate on the incorporation of tritiated precursors in DNA and the thickness of the inter-follicular epidermis, and their relation to tumor promotion in mouse skin. Cancer Res 32: 1562.

Saffiotti, U, Montesano, R, Sellakumar, A, Borg, S (1967). Experimental cancer of the lung: Inhibition by vitamin A of the induction of tracheobronchial squamous metaplasia and squamous cell tumors. Cancer 20: 857.

Schroder, E, Black, P (1980). Retinoids: tumor preventers or tumor enhancers? J Natl Cancer Inst 65: 671.

Silverman, J, Katayama, S, Zelenakas, K, Lauber, J, Musser, T, Reddy, M, Levenstein, M, Weisburger, J (1981). Effect of retinoids on the induction of colon cancer in F344 rats by N-methyl-N-nitrosourea or by 1,2-dimethylhydrazine. Carcinogenesis 2: 1167.

Slaga, T, Fischer, S, Nelson, K, Gleason, G (1980a). Studies on the mechanism of skin tumor promotion: evidence for several stages in promotion. Proc Natl Acad Sci USA 77: 3659.

Slaga, T, Klein-Szanto, A, Fischer, S, Weeks, C, Nelson, K, Major, S (1980b). Studies of mechanism of action of anti-tumor-promoting agents: their specificity in two-stage promotion. Proc Natl Acad Sci USA 77: 2251.

Solanki, V and Slaga, T (1981). Specific binding of phorbol ester tumor promoters to intact primary epidermal cells from SENCAR mice. Proc Natl Acad Sci USA 78: 2549.

Sporn, M B, Newton, D (1981). Retinoids and chemoprevention of cancer. In Zedeck, M, Lipkin, M (eds.) "Inhibition of Tumor Induction and Development," New York: Plenum, p.71.

Sporn, M, Squire, R, Brown, C, Smith, J, Wenk, M L, Springer, S (1977). 13-cis-Retinoic acid: inhibition of bladder carcinogenesis in the rat. Science 195: 487.

Stinson, S, Reznik, G, Donahoe, R (1981). Effect of three retinoids on tracheal carcinogenesis with N-methyl-N-nitrosourea in hamsters. J Natl Cancer Inst 66: 947.

Verma, A (1981). Biochemical mechanism of modulation of skin carcinogenesis by retinoids. In. C.E. Orfanos (ed): "Retinoids," Springer-Verlag, p.117.

Verma, A, Boutwell, R (1977). Vitamin A acid (retinoic acid), a potent inhibitor of 12-0-tetradecanoyl-phorbol-13-acetate-induced ornithine decarboxylase activity in mouse epidermis. Cancer Res 37: 2196.

Verma, A, Conrad, E, Boutwell, R (1980). Induction of mouse epidermal ornithine decarboxylase activity and skin tumors by 7,12-dimethylbenz[a]anthracene: modulation by retinoic acid and 7,8-benzoflavone. Carcinogenesis 1: 607.

Verma, A, Conrad, E, Boutwell, R (1982). Differential effects of retinoic acid and 7,8-benzoflavone on the induction of mouse skin tumors by the complete carcinogenesis process and by the initiation-promotion regimen. Cancer Res 42: 3519.

Verma, A, Rice, H, Shapas, B, Boutwell, R (1978). Inhibition of 12-0-tetradecanoylphorbol-13-acetate-induced ornithine decarboxylase activity in mouse epidermis by vitamin A analogs (retinoids). Cancer Res 38: 793.

Verma, A, Shapas, B, Rice, H, Boutwell, R (1979). Correlation of the inhibition by retinoids of tumor promoter-induced mouse epidermal ornithine decarboxylase activity and of skin tumor promotion. Cancer Res 39: 419.

Welsch, C., Goodrich-Smith, M., Brown, C., Crowe, N. (1981). Enhancement by retinyl acetate of hormone-induced mammary tumorigenesis in female GR/A mice. J Natl Cancer Inst 67: 935.

Yuspa, S H (1981-1982). Chemical carcinogenesis related to the skin. Prog Dermatol 15: 1, 16: 1.

Yuspa, S H, Ben, T, Hennings, H, Lichti, U (1980a). Phorbol ester tumor promoters induce epidermal transglutaminase activity. Biochem Biophy Res Commun 97: 700.

Yuspa, S H, Ben, T, Hennings, H, Lichti, U (1982a). Divergent responses in epidermal basal cells exposed to the tumor promoter 12-0-tetradecanoylphorbol-13-acetate. Cancer Res 42: 2344.

Yuspa, S H, Ben, T, Steinert, P (1982b). Retinoic acid induces transglutaminase activity but inhibits cornification of cultured epidermal cells. J Biol Chem, in press.

Yuspa, S H, Harris, C C (1982). Molecular and cellular basis of chemical carcinogenesis. In Schottenfeld, D and Fraumeni, J (eds.): "Cancer Epidemiology and Prevention," Philadelphia: W B Saunders, p. 23.

Yuspa, S H, Hawley-Nelson, P, Stanley, J, Hennings, H (1980b). Epidermal cell culture. Transplant Proc 12, Suppl 1: 114.

Yuspa, S H, Hennings, H, Lichti, U (1981a). Initiator and promoter induced specific changes in epidermal function and biological potential. J Supramol Struct and Cell Biochem 17: 245.

Yuspa, S H, Lichti, U, Ben, T, Hennings, H (1981b). Modulation of terminal differentiation and responses to tumor promoters by retinoids in mouse epidermal cell cultures. Ann NY Acad Sci 359: 260.

Yuspa, S H, Morgan, D (1981). Mouse skin cells resistant to terminal differentiation associated with initiation of carcinogenesis. Nature 293: 72.

Diet, Nutrition, and Cancer:
From Basic Research to Policy Implications, pages 111–115
© *1983 Alan R. Liss, Inc., 150 Fifth Avenue, New York, NY 10011*

DEFICIENCY OF VITAMIN A IN HEPATOCELLULAR CARCINOMA TISSUE:
CONSIDERATIONS ON ITS ESTABLISHMENT

Luigi M. De Luca, Ph.D.

Differentiation Control Section
National Cancer Institute
Bethesda, MD 20205

Dietary components, whether beneficial or toxic, represent the major source of body tissue constituents. Therefore,
it is only reasonable to expect that some of the food components may partake in the complex interactions, which eventually lead to the development of cancer or its prevention.

Mutagens, complete carcinogens, as well as tumor promoting substances are present in the diet, and intake of such
compounds may be limited by consumption of selected foods,
by proper food storage techniques as well as by the preferen-
tial utilization of certain procedures for the preparation of
foods, which may minimize the production of mutagenic agents.

However, it is becoming increasingly clear that even the
most careful and well informed individual may not escape
exposure to mutagens, carcinogens and tumor promoters in the
diet or as inhaled in the respiratory system or absorbed
through the skin. Therefore it becomes important to consider
that the diet is also the source of beneficial substances,
which may function as preventive agents of carcinogenesis.
Recent evidence suggests that eating a diet rich in vegetables
and fiber may protect the individual against the development
of certain cancers (Modan et al., 1975; Bjelke, 1975; Reddy
et al., 1980). Specifically the work of Wattenberg (1980)
has stressed the concept that naturally occurring substances
may function as preventive agents of chemical carcinogenesis
and epidemiological evidence lends support to this concept
(Doll and Peto, 1981).

Essential nutrient deficiency and tumor development. The essential nutrient vitamin A and its provitamins (Peto et al., 1981) have also been implicated as tumor preventing substances in the process of carcinogenesis. The most convincing evidence that physiological levels of vitamin A are protective against the development of cancer comes from the work of Cone and Nettesheim (1973), who demonstrated that the condition of vitamin A deficiency may act as a permissive factor in the development of 3-methyl-cholanthrene induced lung cancer. The work of Bollag (1972), Sporn and Newton (1979), and others (reviewed by De Luca, 1978) has tended to support the concept that doses of vitamin A above physiological levels protect the animal from the development of epithelial cancer. Therefore it can be argued that, if the condition of vitamin A deficiency represents one of the permissive factors in tumor development, the maintenance of the deficiency state may be required for the tumor cell to continue as a tumor.

If this were true, a mechanism should exist to create a cell for which the nutrient is no longer essential, and which can in fact thrive under conditions of deficiency of the essential nutrient or of one of its functions; such conditions would not be compatible with differentiation and growth of normal cells. This hypothesis expects that the condition of essential nutrient deficiency should be quite common in neoplastic cells. In a study of the vitamin A content of hepatocellular carcinoma cell microsomal membranes compared to the host liver, we could not find detectable amounts of retinyl palmitate in ten transplanted Morris hepatomas, while normal ranges of concentrations were found in the host liver microsomes (De Luca et al., 1982). In other words the hepatomas appeared to be in a status similar to that of vitamin A depleted liver, which indicates that the hepatoma cells are independent of vitamin A for their function.

The microsomes from the hepatoma tissue also contained 50 to 100% less of the phosphorylated vitamin A than the host, resembling the situation of vitamin A deficient liver tissue.

However there are obvious differences between vitamin A depleted liver and the hepatoma tissue. First the inability of the latter to become repleted in the presence of ample pools of the vitamin and secondly the tendency of the tumor tissue to survive and proliferate, while the vitamin A deficient tissue eventually ceases to grow.

Tumor phenotype as a consequence of essential nutrient
deficiency status. It should be considered that the condition
of vitamin A deficiency in the respiratory tract of rodents
causes the replacement of the normally mucociliary epithelium
by a squamous metaplastic epithelium, similar to the skin
(Yuspa et al., 1982). It becomes then interesting to consider
that the most common type of lung cancer, though presumably
(but not certainly) arising from a mucosecretory or ciliated
cell, displays a squamous metaplastic phenotype similar to
that of the vitamin A deficient cell of the respiratory tract
(Harris et al., 1972). It should also be considered that the
tumor promoter 12-0-tetradecanoyl-phorbol-13-acetate (TPA)
acts on non-initiated cells by accelerating the squamous
keratinizing type of differentiation in cultured mouse
epidermal cells (Yuspa et al., 1982).

Tumor promotion as a result of essential nutrient deficiency in initiated cells. Based on these considerations, I
would like to propose 1. that tumor promoting substances
(e.g. TPA) may act by causing a localized condition of deficiency of the physiological antipromoter (e.g. vitamin A) or
of the expression of its function; 2. that non-initiated cells
respond to such deficiency condition by either differentiating
and dying off, as is the case for the epidermal cells, or by
inhibition of growth and cell death; 3. that the essential
nutrient inhibits the expression of the mutation present in
the initiated cells; and 4. that the initiated cell under conditions of essential nutrient deficiency adapts and prevails
by expressing a phenotype, which is characteristic of the
deficiency condition. Such phenotype confers a growth advan-
advantage to the initiated cell, because it has arisen as the
expression of a mutation maintained dormant by the essential
nutrient (or its function) under normal conditions.

In this program of events the presence of the mutation in
initiated cells, while by itself incapable of expressing the
tumorigenic phenotype because of the counteracting action of
the physiological antipromoter, allows such expression by
creating an adapted phenotype, which does not need the essential nutrient for survival. It would then follow that the
tumor cell would find itself in a status of greater nutritional antonomy at least for that essential nutrient, the
deficiency of which was responsible in the very beginning
for the expression of the tumor from initiated cells. The
cell then would survive under conditions which would not
permit the growth of normal cells.

This hypothesis may explain the variety of phenotypes in tumors arising from the same tissue, depending on the particular expression resulting from deficiency of the specific antipromoter as caused by the promoting substance. Therefore the following concepts should be addressed:

1. Certain essential nutrients or substances which control proper differentiation are of the utmost importance for maintaining mutated (initiated) cells in the dormant (non-expressed) state.

2. Conditions of localized deficiency of essential nutrients, whether caused by foreign chemicals, radiation, xenobiotics or excess of other nutrients which consume the essential element for their own metabolism, should be avoided by proper dietary habits or, when defective transport mechanisms are identified, by utilizing the form of the essential nutrient which bypasses normal transport (e.g. retinoic acid instead of retinol).

3. The combination of chemical additives, such as artificial or natural substances, with which the body has not come in contact in the diet in its evolution, may present a considerable metabolic burden and may function as a tumor promoting stimulus by exhausting the supply of essential nutrients.

A conservative policy of consuming traditional foods without excessive and unnecessary burdens of artificial colors and flavors should be followed whenever possible.

Bjelke E (1975). Dietary vitamin A and human lung cancer. Int J Cancer 15:561.

Bollag W (1972). Prophilaxis of chemically induced benign and malignant epithelial tumors by vitamin A acid (retinoic acid). Eur J Cancer 8:689.

Cone MV and Nettesheim P (1973). Effects of vitamin A on 3-methyl cholanthrene-induced squamous metaplasias and early tumors in the respiratory tract of rats. J Natl Cancer Inst 50:1599.

De Luca LM (1978). Vitamin A, in De Luca HF (ed): "Handbook of lipid research", Vol. 2, New York: Plenum Publishing Corporation, p 1.

De Luca LM, Brugh M, Silverman-Jones CS (1982). Submitted for publication.

Doll R, Peto R (1981). The causes of cancer: Quuantitative estimates of avoidable risks of cancer in the United States today. J Natl Cancer Inst 66:1191.

Modan B, Barell V, Lubin F et al. (1975). Low-fiber intake as an etiologic factor in cancer of the colon. J Natl Cancer Inst 55:15.

Harris CC, Sporn MB, Kaufman DG et al. (1972). Histogenesis of squamous metaplasia in the hamster tracheal epithelium caused by vitamin A deficiency or benzo[a]pyrene ferric oxide. J Natl Cancer Inst 48:743.

Peto R, Doll R, Buckley JD et al. (1981). Can dietary beta-carotene materially reduce human cancer rates. Nature 290:201.

Sporn MB, Newton DC (1979). Chemoprevention of cancer with retinoids. Fed Proc 38:2528

Wattenberg LW (1980). Inhibitors of chemical carcinogenesis. J Environ Pathol Toxicol 3:35.

Yuspa SH, Ben T, Hennings H and Lichti U (1982). Divergent responses in epidermal basal cells exposed to the tumor promoter 12-0-tetradecanoyl-13-acetate. Cancer Res 42:2344.

Diet, Nutrition, and Cancer:
From Basic Research to Policy Implications, pages 117–123
© *1983 Alan R. Liss, Inc., 150 Fifth Avenue, New York, NY 10011*

RETINOIDS, CELLULAR RETINOID BINDING PROTEINS, NUCLEUS,
AND CANCER

F. Chytil, M. Omori, G. Liau and D. E. Ong

Department of Biochemistry
Vanderbilt University School of Medicine
Nashville, TN 37232

Recent years have brought hard evidence that vitamin
A status and vitamin A metabolism are of interest in malignant growth (Sporn et al. 1976). However even as early
as 1922 a vitamin A-deficient diet was used in the unsuccess-
ful treatment of cancer patients (Wyard 1922). Later,
Wolbach and Howe (1925) pointed out the similarity of
morphological changes caused by vitamin A deficiency to
the morphology of some cancers. These authors observed,
in many tissues, that vitamin A deficiency resulted in
the replacement of normal columnar and transitional epithelium by squamous, frequently keratinizing epithelial cells.
These tissues of the vitamin A deficient rat had a high
mitotic index and the authors concluded that the behavior
of the cells indicated a growth power suggestive of neoplastic potentiality (Wolbach and Howe 1925). However these
metaplastic changes can be reversed by refeeding the animal
with the nutrient (Wolbach and Howe 1933).

It has now become evident that vitamin A deficient
animals are more susceptible to some carcinogenic insults
(Davies 1967; Rowe et al. 1970; Nettesheim and Williams
1976). In some cases however vitamin A deficient animals
have developed significantly fewer carcinogen-induced
epithelial metaplasias and tumors (Narisawa et al 1976).
Consequently the experimental evidence suggests that vitamin
A deficiency may permit a higher incidence of some tumors
in some experimental systems but may inhibit development
of other types of cancer in other test systems. Similarly
pharmacological amounts of vitamin A have been shown to
inhibit (Saffioti et al. 1967; Bollag 1970) or potentiate

the effect of carcinogens (Schroder and Black 1980).
These facts should be kept in mind when one attempts to
analyze how vitamin A like compounds exert their action
in the normal and malignant cells on the molecular level.
Efforts to elucidate molecular mechanisms in vitamin A
action indifferentiation of epithelia as well as its effects
on malignant growth have produced little success at this
point.

Two compounds of the vitamin A family are of particular
interest, all-trans retinol, provided by the diet, and
retinoic acid, a natural metabolite of retinol. Retinol,
as well as esters and ethers of retinol, and retinoic
acid as well as various synthetic analogues of the acid
have shown promise as prophylactic and therapeutic agents
against spontaneous and chemically induced tumors (Bollag
1970; Sporn et al 1976; Mayer et al. 1978).

We believe that in order to understand effects of
retinoids on malignant growth it will be necessary to
understand how these compounds regulate differentiation
of normal tissues. Our laboratory has been involved in
elucidation of the molecular mechanisms of vitamin A action.
We have assumed that the cell nucleus and its metabolic
machinery is responsible for cell differentiation. This
working hypothesis led us to explore possible specific
interactions of retinol or retinoic acid with the cell
nucleus. Such interactions of retinol or retinoic acid
with the nucleus should lead to alterations in genomic
expression. We believe that the results of this approach
could help elucidate the molecular mechanisms which operate
during normal as well as malignant growth. Indeed considerable evidence has been accumulated in the past showing
that the cell nucleus and gene expression is altered in
malignancy (Koller 1963).

Two intracellular retinoic binding proteins exist
in many tissues. both have been isolated and partially
characterized (Bashor et al. 1973; Ong and Chytil 1975;
Chytil and Ong 1978, 1979). The first is cellular retinol-
binding protein (CRBP); the second is cellular retinoic
acid-binding protein (CRABP). CRBP binds retinol with
high specificity and affinity, but does not bind retinal
or retinoic acid. It carries retinol in vivo (Ong and
Chytil 1975; Ong et al 1976). CRABP has high affinity
for retinoic acid but does not bind retinol or retinal.

Recently it has been shown that it carries retinoic acid
in vivo (Saari et al 1982). The levels of these proteins
change during perinatal development in a nonsynchronous
manner (Ong and Chytil 1976a). It appears that the genes
coding for those proteins are turned on and off during
normal growth. Considerable evidence has been accumulated
by workers of many laboratories that the levels of these
cellular retinoid binding proteins also change during
malignant growth, suggesting that the genomic expression
of these proteins undergoes alterations in malignancy
(Ong et al. 1975, 1978, 1982; Ong and Chytil 1976b see
also reviews; Chytil and Ong 1978, 1982a,b). Parenthetical-
ly no structural or binding differences have been observed
in these proteins when they were studied in normal and
malignant tissues (Chytil and Ong 1976).

We have studied the mode of interaction of CRBP and
retinol within the cell nucleus. We have reported previously that purified cellular retinol-binding protein (CRBP)
will mediate specific binding of retinol to nuclei isolated
from rat liver (Takase et al. 1979). We have recently
found that pure CRBP delivers retinol to the specific
nuclear binding sites without itself remaining bound.
Triton X-100-treated nuclei retain the majority of these
binding sites. CRBP is also capable of delivering retinol
specifically to isolated chromatin with no apparent loss
of binding sites, as compared to whole nuclei. CRBP again
does not remain bound after transferring retinol to the
chromatin binding sites. When isolated nuclei are incubated
with [^{3}H]retinol-CRBP, sectioned, and autoradiographed,
specifically bound retinol is found distributed throughout
the nuclei. Thus, CRBP delivers retinol to the interior
of the nucleus, to specific binding sites which are primarily, if not solely, on the chromatin (Liau et al. 1981).
Interaction of retinol with these specific binding sites
may alter structure and function of chromatin which in
turn results in altered gene expression. Whether and
how CRBP interacts with nuclei from cancer cells remains
to be elucidated.

Recently we have attempted to look at the possible
changes which might occur in gene expression of vitamin
A deficient animals (Omori and Chytil, 1982). The effects
of retinol and retinoic acid on genomic expression were
studied in rat testis, intestinal mucosa and liver by
determining total cytoplasmic poly(A)-containing RNA,

by using techniques of molecular hybridization and in
vitro translation. Dietary retinol deficiency induces
loss of poly(A)-containing RNA in all tissues studied.
Homologous and heterologous hybridization of poly(A)-con-
taining RNAs from testes of retinol deficient and control
rats to complementary DNAs (cDNAs) showed differences
especially in the fast annealing sequences, which are
expressed in smaller quantities in retinol deficient rats.
Polyacrylamide gel electrophoresis and subsequent fluorogra-
phy of in vitro translation of cytoplasmic poly(A)-contain-
ing RNA revealed additional and more intensive bands repre-
senting polypeptides in the region of 15,000 and 27,000
Daltons when testicular preparations from deficient rats
were compared with those from controls. One hour after
feeding of retinol deficient rats with retinylacetate
as source of retinol, a loss of poly(A)-containing RNA
in testicular and intestinal mucosa is observed. Subsequently this RNA accumulates, but does not reach control levels
even after refeeding with the vitamin for two weeks.
The fast reaction of the genomic expression is also evident,
when patterns of in vitro translation products are analyzed
in testicular preparations. One hour after dosing deficient
animals with retinyl acetate, retinoic acid or a synthetic
derivative of retinoic acid, a polypeptide band of 22,000
Daltons disappears. When retinoic acid, or a synthetic
derivative of retinoic acid is administered in contrast
to retinylacetate a band of 55,000 Daltons intensifies.
The data indicate that retinol and retinoic acid influence
genomic expression in vivo by activation as well as by
simultaneous suppression of the genome. Moreover, it
appears that the effects of retinol and retinoic acid
are rapid and not identical.

Further work is necessary to characterize the gene
products influenced by retinoids. Moreover it will be
necessary to find out whether and how retinoids change
genomic expression in various tumors. Experiments are
now in progress in our laboratory to establish whether
the cellular binding proteins are involved functionally
in genomic expression of normal and malignant tissue.

ACKNOWLEDGEMENTS

The work of the authors was supported by USPHS grant
HD-09195 from the National Institute for Child and Human

Development, grant CA-20850 from the National Cancer Institute and grants HL-14214, HL-15341 from the National Heart, Lung and Blood Institute.

REFERENCES

Bashor MM, Toft DE, Chytil F (1973). In vitro binding of retinol to rat-tissue components. Proc Natl Acad Sci USA 70:3483.

Bollag W (1970). Vitamin A and vitamin A acid in the prophylaxis and therapy of epithelial tumors. Int J Vit Nutr Res 40:299.

Chytil F, Ong DE (1976). Mediation of retinoic acid induced growth and anti-tumour activity. Nature 260:5546.

Chytil F, Ong DE (1978). Cellular vitamin A binding proteins. Vitam Horm 36:1.

Chytil F, Ong DE (1979). Cellular retinol and retinoic acid-binding proteins in vitamin A action. Fed Proc 38:2510.

Chytil F, Ong DE (1982a). Retinoid binding proteins and human cancer. In Arnott MS, van Eyes J, Wang YM (eds): "Molecular Interrelations of Nutrition and Cancer", New York: Raven Press, p 409.

Chytil F, Ong DE (1982b). Cellular retinol and retinoic acid binding proteins. In Draper HH (ed): "Advances in Nutritional Research", vol , New York: Plenum Press, in Press.

Davies DE (1967). Effect of vitamin A on 7,12-dimethyl-benz(a)anthracene-induced papillomas in rhino mouse skin. Cancer Res 27:237.

Koller PC (1963). The nucleus of the cancer cell. A historical review. Exp Cell Res Suppl 9:3.

Liau G, Ong DE, Chytil F (1981). Interaction of the retinol/cellular retinol-binding protein complex with isolated nuclei and nuclear components. J Cell Biol 91:63.

Mayer H, Bollag W, Hänni R, Rüegg R (1978). Retinoids, a new class of compounds with prophylactic and therapeutic activities in oncology and dermatology. Experientia 34:1105.

Narisawa T, Reddy BS, Wong CO, Weisburger JH (1976). Effect of vitamin A deficiency on rat colon carcinogenesis by N'methyl-N'-nitro-N-nitroso-guanidine. Cancer Res 36:1379.

Nettesheim P, Williams ML (1976). The influence of vitamin A on the susceptibility of the rat lung to 3-methylcholan-threne. Int J Cancer 17:351.

Omori M, Chytil F (1982). Mechanism of vitamin A action: Gene expression in retinol deficient rats. J Biol Chem in Press.

Ong DE, Chytil F (1975). Retinoic acid binding protein in rat tissue. J Biol Chem 250:6113.

Ong DE, Chytil F (1976a). Changes in levels of cellular retinol- and retinoic-acid-binding proteins of liver and lung during perinatal development of rat. Proc Natl Acad Sci USA 73:3976.

Ong DE, Chytil F (1976b). Presence of cellular retinol and retinoic acid binding proteins in experimental tumors. Cancer Lett 2:25.

Ong DE, Page DL, Chytil F (1975). Retinoic acid binding protein: Occurrence in human tumors. Science 190:60.

Ong DE, Tsai CH, Chytil F (1976). Cellular retinol-binding protein and retinoic acid-binding protein in rat testes: effect of retinol depletion. J Nutr 106:204.

Ong DE, Markert C, Chiu JF (1978). Cellular binding proteins for vitamin A in colorectal adenocarcinoma of rat. Cancer Res 38:4422.

Ong DE, Goodwin WJ, Jesse RH, Griffin AC (1982). Presence of cellular retinol and retinoic acid-binding proteins in epidermoid carcinoma of the oral cavity and oropharynx. Cancer 49:1409.

Rowe NH, Grammer FC, Watson FR, Nickerson NH (1970). A study of environmental influence upon salivary gland neoplasia in rats. Cancer 26:436.

Saari JC, Bredberg L, Garwin G (1982). Endogenous retinoids associated with three cellular retinoic-binding proteins from bovine retina. Fed Proc 41:861.

Saffiotti U, Montesano R, Sellakumar AR, Borg SA (1967). Experimental cancer of the lung. Inhibition by vitamin A of the induction of tracheobronchial squamous metapla-sia and squamous cell tumors. Cancer 20:857.

Schroder EW, Black PH (1980). Retinoids: Tumor prevent-ers or tumor enhancers? J Natl Cancer Inst USA 65:671.

Sporn MB, Dunlop NM, Newton DL, Smith JM (1976). Preven-tion of chemical carcinogenesis by vitamin A and its synthetic analogs (retinoids). Fed Proc 35:1332.

Takase S, Ong DE, Chytil F (1979). Cellular retinol-bind-ing protein allows specific interaction of retinol with the nucleus in vitro. Proc Natl Acad Sci USA 76:2204.

Wolbach SB, Howe PR (1925). Tissue changes following deprivation of fat-soluble A vitamin. J Exp Med 42:753.
Wolbach SB, Howe PR (1933). Epithelial repair in recovery from vitamin A deficiency. J Exp Med 57:511.
Wyard S (1922). The treatment of malignant disease by a diet free from fat-soluble vitamin A. Lancet 202:840.

Diet, Nutrition, and Cancer:
From Basic Research to Policy Implications, pages 125–134
© *1983 Alan R. Liss, Inc., 150 Fifth Avenue, New York, NY 10011*

THE DEVELOPMENT OF RESEARCH ON THE EPIDEMIOLOGY OF VITAMIN
A AND CANCER

Curtis Mettlin, Ph.D.

Director, Cancer Control & Epidemiology
Roswell Park Memorial Institute
Buffalo, New York 14263

INTRODUCTION

The purposes of this report are to describe some of
the epidemiologic evidence that associates vitamin A intake
with reductions in cancer risk, to consider the strengths
and limitations of these data as they relate to public
health policy, and to suggest some future avenues for
epidemiologic research in this field. The scope of this
review is limited to the realm of epidemiologic inquiry
and, of all of the research on vitamin A, epidemiologic
research is the most recent. The first laboratory investigation dates to 1925 (Wolbach and Howe, 1925) but the first
epidemiologic study was not reported until fifty years
later (Bjelke, 1975). Given the recency of this topic as
one of interest to cancer epidemiologists, it is understand-
able that the tools of research are not well refined and
that interpretations of the significance of the limited
available evidence may not be wholly agreed upon.

In spite of some of the controversies that concern
epidemiologic studies of vitamin A and cancer, this type of
inquiry is important for several reasons. First, there are
few, if any, biological universals. Data from in vitro and
animal studies may or may not be pertinent to the human
situation. Epidemiologic studies, by definition, concern
the experience of human populations and are, for this
reason, most relevant to public health. Second, laboratory
studies measure the effects of pure or, at least, refined
substances, whereas epidemiologic studies measure the
effects of exposures as they actually and imperfectly occur

in the environment. Finally, laboratory investigations
rely on intensive levels of exposure which are difficult
to extrapolate to levels which are realistic for humans.
Epidemiologic studies, in contrast, observe exposures at
levels which populations commonly experience. Thus, in
general, the precision of experimental and laboratory
research is obtained at the expense of information on
public health significance. The reverse is true as well.
Epidemiologic studies yield information relevant to human
experience at the expense of the control of confounding
variables and precision of measurement obtainable in the
laboratory. In the best of worlds, in vivo, in vitro and
epidemiologic methods will complement one another. The
study of the relationship between vitamin A and cancer risk
may be one of those uncommon instances where this is the
case and this in itself is important information.

EPIDEMIOLOGIC STUDIES

    The following represents a selective review of studies
associating vitamin A intake to cancer risk. Its purpose
is to illustrate the range and type of data currently available. For a more complete discussion of these and other
studies, the reader is referred to reviews such as those of
Mettlin (1982) or Peto et al. (1980).

    One possible means of assessing the effect of vitamin
A in human carcinogenesis is by comparison of levels of
retinol and/or beta carotene in the blood of cancer patients
to those levels observed in healthy persons or persons
having diseases other than cancer. Ibrahim et al. (1977)
studied blood levels of retinol and beta carotene in 203
Indian patients with squamous cell carcinoma of the oral
cavity and oral pharynx and in 112 control persons matched
for age and sex. They found the cancer patients to have
significantly lower levels of both of these measured
attributes. Lambert et al. (1981) found carotene levels to
be somewhat higher than the serum of in situ carcinoma of
the cervix patients compared to patients with no cancer.
Retinol levels were somewhat lower. The differences were
not statistically significant and the small sample observed
lends the study too little statistical power to conclude one
way or the other with respect to the role of vitamin A in
cervical cancer. Basu et al. (1976) obtained blood samples
from 28 histologically confirmed cases of bronchial carcinoma,

10 healthy subjects, and a patient with non-malignant bronchial disease. For each blood specimen, the level of plasma vitamin A was assessed by laboratory analysis. Cases had significantly lower plasma vitamin A levels than controls although their report is unclear as to the degree the cases and controls were matched for smoking status.

Two studies have been conducted where blood was available from large numbers of persons among whom diagnoses of cancer occurred several years later. In England, serum samples were collected from a population of 16,000 men and stored (Wald et al., 1980). After five years, 86 of these subjects were identified as having developed cancer. Retinol levels in the blood samples of these men and of 172 persons from the population who did not develop cancer were assayed. Low retinol levels were associated with an increased risk of cancer. Overall, a 2.2-fold increase in risk was observed comparing men in the highest quintile to those in the lowest.

Using a similar design, Kark et al. (1981) followed 3,102 men from Evans County, Georgia for 12 to 14 years. Blood samples had been obtained from these men as part of their participation in a prospective study of coronary heart disease risk factors. The subsequent documented finding of 129 cases of cancer in the population made it possible to study the relationship of serum retinol levels and cancer risk in this population. Persons who had eventually developed cancer were found to have had significantly lower mean serum retinol levels at least 12 months prior to the cancer diagnosis.

Vitamin A levels in the blood may or not accurately reflect dietary exposure to vitamin A. Another vein of research, therefore, is that which attempts to measure dietary intake of vitamin A in patients and control subjects. Bjelke (1975) reported the results of a five year prospective study of 8,278 Norwegian men who reported their cigarette smoking and dietary habits by mailed survey. Among these men, 36 cases of bronchus carcinoma were identified by means of the Norway Cancer Registry. An index of vitamin A intake was obtained by weighting the frequency respondents reported consuming several food items by the vitamin A content of a standard portion of each and, summing the products. Bjelke found a significant negative association between the vitamin index and cancer mortality at all levels of cigarette smoking.

MacLennan et al. (1977) studied the high incidence of lung cancer among the Chinese population of Singapore. Several questions were asked regarding frequency of consumption of common dark green leafy vegetables such as Chinese mustard greens and kale. This research showed a 2.23-fold increase in risk associated with relatively low frequency of consumption of these dark green leafy vegetables.

During a period from 1954 to 1965, all patients entering Roswell Park Memorial Institute in Buffalo, New York, were interviewed with respect to their usual dietary habits. A measure of vitamin intake was obtained from questions regarding the patients' usual frequency of consumption of 21 different food items during the months one year prior to the onset of symptoms (Mettlin et al., 1979). The vitamin A content of the diet was estimated by U.S. Department of Agriculture tables of food values for a standard portion of each item. The products of this weighting factor and the monthly frequency consumption were summed for all food items. The dietary interview did not examine all the foods that might be eaten by the respondents and the vitamin A index was an estimate of relative, rather than absolute, vitamin A intake based on a substantial portion of food ingestion. The age and smoking-adjusted relative risks for varying levels of vitamin A intake showed descending levels of risk associated with ascending levels of the vitamin A index with a 2.4-fold reduction in risk for the highest level of vitamin A. Milk and carrots, common sources of dietary vitamin A, contributed significantly to the overall vitamin A index and these were the only food items that, independent of the index, were associated with lung cancer risk. Elevated risks were observed for persons who reported typically drinking less than one, as opposed to greater than one, cup of milk per day. Carrot consumption was associated with reduced lung cancer risks but only among the heavy smoking men. Among the lighter smokers or non-smokers, there was no differentiation in risk associated with the frequency of carrot consumption.

Our study of 569 bladder cancer patients and 1,025 age matched controls admitted to Roswell Park (Mettlin and Graham, 1980) showed sex-adjusted relative risks increased at lower levels of vitamin A intake measured in the same fashion as was done in the lung cancer study. A similar pattern of risk elevation was associated with infrequent milk and carrot intake.

The Roswell Park data have also shown relationships between vitamin A intake and relative risk of laryngeal cancer (Graham et al., 1981) and oral cancer (Marshall et al., 1982). No reduction of risk was observed for colon and rectum cancer (Graham et al., 1978). Recently, we reported evidence of elevation of breast cancer risk associated with lower levels of vitamin A exposure as measured by the Roswell Park diet interview (Graham et al., 1982). The levels of risk were not markedly high (RR = 1.4) and were not uniform across groups of different risk status as measured by age. Statistical significance however, was attainable due to the rather large number of cases studied. Studies of other sites from these data remain to be reported.

The original Roswell Park study of vitamin A in lung cancer has been replicated in England by Gregor et al., (1981). They obtained estimates of current dietary vitamin A intake from 100 lung cancer cases and 173 controls. Patients were interviewed regarding their current patterns of consumption of major dietary sources of vitamin A including cheese, eggs, butter, margarine, milk, liver, carrots, green vegetables as well as regarding their use of vitamin pills. They found total current vitamin A intake to be particularly lower in male lung cancer cases than in comparable control patients. Marked differences were observed between cases and controls with respect to their consumption of liver and of vitamin A supplements. Vitamin A intake from liver was significantly lower in male lung cancer patients than in controls although this was not found to be true for females, where the lung cancer cases reported higher intake of vitamin A via liver consumption than did age-matched controls.

The researchers of the Western Electric Study examined their data to determine the 19 year incidence of lung cancer among 1,954 middle-aged men. Thirty-three men in this population were observed to have developed lung cancer three to nineteen years after they had been interviewed with respect to their dietary habits. Their vitamin A intake was classified as to the degree it was "preformed" vitamin A (retinol) or, carotene. Shekelle et al., (1981) reported that fourteen of 488 men estimated to have the lowest level of carotene intake developed lung cancer and only two of an equal number in the highest quartile of carotene exposure were so diagnosed. For no cancer other than lung did the carotene or retinol index significantly deviate from the values observed for the study population as a whole.

Hirayama (1976) reporting a ten-year prospective study of 256,118 Japanese adults, found associations between the frequency of green and yellow vegetable consumption and rates of mortality from lung cancer. Among both males and females, regardless of smoking habits, persons who reported daily consumption of green and yellow vegetables had significantly lower rates of lung cancer mortality than those who reported occasional or less frequent consumption of these food items.

DISCUSSION

Although the hypothesis that exposure to vitamin A can reduce cancer risk may be seen as supported by a significant body of epidemiologic evidence, enthusiasm for the hypothesis should not be untempered. It is the nature of science that positive associations will be reported first in the litera- ture. Contrary findings or failure to find any association are just now becoming interesting research outcomes and increased reporting of negative studies may be in the offing. This is particularly possible in light of the fact that few of the investigations reported to date were designed to test the hypothesis that exposure to vitamin A affects human cancer risk. With a few exceptions such as Gregor's study, epidemiologic studies of vitamin A and cancer have relied on secondary analysis of data originally being collected for other purposes. In most cases, the procedures and measures relied upon were not those that would be chosen were one to design a study and collect data specifically to test the hypothesis. For example, the Roswell Park data does not include information on eggs, liver, vitamin tablet and other sources of vitamin A that we wished had been obtained. In the case of the Western Electric Study, the data which would provide a more accurate measure of retinol as opposed to carotene were no longer available and an index procedure of unknown validity had to be employed. Future investigations, focusing particularly on this question, may provide more reliable information than the largely serendipitous epidemi- ologic studies to date.

A question that cannot be resolved by examination of published data is whether different types of sources of vitamin A confer different levels of risk modification. For example, Peto et al., (1981) contend on theoretical grounds that beta-carotene rather than retinol would be the more effective agent in reducing risk. However, the evidence from multiple studies is that several non-carotene sources of vitamin A such as liver, milk and vitamin A containing preparations are associated with reduced risk of cancer at different sites. Our studies of lung and bladder cancer, for example, showed that milk, a potential source of retinol vitamin A in the typical American diet, was associated with reduced risk and in the Gregor study of lung cancer, only the retinol sources were associated with risk reduction. These findings are contradicted only by the Western Electric Study and there, the original data on intake are unavailable. In addition, the large majority of animal studies which suggest a protective effect from vitamin A used a retinoid to induce the observed effects. Thus, the available evidence from human populations does not compel one to conclude one way or the other concerning this question. Obviously, this is an issue for future research.

From a public health perspective, however, this may not be that significant a question. Just as we are sure of the benefits of avoiding exposure to cigarettes without knowing the precise properties of cigarettes which make them so harmful, we may come to a knowledge that exposure to certain foods confers protective effects without ever learning what precise biochemical properties of those foods are responsible for the benefits derived.

Because the acceptance of a preventive measure by the population at risk is an important variable in the implementation of cancer control measure (Graham, 1964, Mettlin, 1979), it may be prudent at this time to consider the characteristics of populations to whom dietary intervention is acceptable. If persons at high risk of disease are least likely to comply with a recommended regimens, this may suggest the need for greater public education directed toward those high risk groups. It would be valuable also to learn whether smokers who wish to pursue the possibility of dietary change are persons who have already attempted smoking cessation and have failed or whether dietary change is most appealing to persons who have not been motivated to smoking cessation. At present, the risk characteristics of persons likely to comply and those of persons unlikely to comply are unknown.

Additionally, at the present, there are no tools at the disposal of cancer control researchers to provide assessments of risk status relative to the need. Such tools will be necessary to identify persons for whom intervention may be appropriate and to monitor adherence to a regimen. A concise questionnaire may be suitable to the risk of identifying candidates for intervention and for monitoring compliance with recommendations. Persons who have levels of dietary intake of natural inhibitors may be differentiated from those who do not, persons who are willing and capable of the behavior changes required may be identified, and persons whose risk status justifies preventive intervention may be located within a more general population. It may also be possible to determine who in the population is complying to the prophylactic recommendation and who may require additional follow-up and education with respect to compliance.

The need for such procedures relates to former experience in cancer control and preventive health which shows that, in some instances, persons at highest risk are less likely to pursue preventive medicine practices such as seeking pap smears (Kleinman and Kostein, 1981). Also, experience with the prophylactic trials of penicillin in rheumatic fever reported by Gordis (1969), shows that compliance may be a serious constraint to the ability of the trial research design to demonstrate and effect.

Finally, lung cancer is the cancer site that has been the subject of research most frequently. This is perhaps due to its high incidence and the ease with which sufficient numbers of subjects can be accessioned in to study. While other sites have been investigated, few have been the subject of multiple investigations and particular efforts in extending the research to a range of cancer sites may be advisable. It is conceivable that benefits achieved in reduction of risk for one or a few types of cancer may be balanced by elevations in risk of other cancers or other adverse health effects.

SUMMARY

The available epidemiologic evidence on the effects of vitamin A on cancer risk are encouraging. The suggest it may be possible to lower cancer incidence by dietary and/or pharmacological interventions. There are consistencies among multiple epidemiologic studies and these, in turn, are compatible with animal and in vitro investigations. However, further consideration in the forms of expanded basic and epidemiologic research needs to be directed toward several issues and it remains to be determined whether purposeful intervention is likely to yield improvements in the public's health.

Basu TK, Donaldson D, Jenner M, Williams DC and Sakulu A (1976). Plasma vitamin A in patients with bronchial carcinoma. Brit J Cancer 33:119.

Bjelke E (1975). Dietary vitamin A and human lung cancer. Int J Cancer 15:561.

Gordis L et al (1969). Studies on the epidemiology and preventability of rheumatic fever. IV A quantitative determination of compliance in children on oral penicillin prophylaxis. Pediatrics 43:173-182.

Graham S (1964). Sociological aspects of health and illness. In Faris REL (ed): "Handbook of Modern Sociology", Chicago: Rand McNally & Co, p. 310-357.

Graham S, Dayal H, Swanson M, Mittelman A and Wilkinson G (1978). Diet in the epidemiology of the colon and rectum. J Natl Cancer Inst 61:709.

Graham S, Mettlin C, Marshall J, Priore R, Rzepka T and Shedd D (1981). Dietary factors in the epidemiology of cancer of the larynx. Am J Epidemiol 113:675.

Graham S, Marshall J, Mettlin C, Rzepka T, Nemoto T and Byers T (1982). Diet in the epidemiology of breast cancer. Am J Epidemiol 116:68-75.

Gregor A, Lee PN, Roe FJC, Wilson MJ and Melton A (1980). Comparison of dietary histories in lung cancer cases and controls with special reference to vitamin A. Nutr Cancer 2:93.

Hirayama T (1979). Diet and cancer. Nutr Cancer 1:67.

Ibrahim K, Jafrey NA and Zuberi SJ (1977). Plasma vitamin 'A' and carotene levels in squamous cell carcinoma of oral cavity and oro-pharynx. Clin Oncology 3:203.

Kark JD, Smith AH, Switzer BR and Hanes CG (1981). Serum vitamin A (retinol) and cancer incidence in Evans County, Georgia. J Natl Cancer Inst 66:7.

Kleinman JC and Kostein A (1981). Who is being screened for cervical cancer? Am J Pub Health 71:59-62.

Lambert B, Brisson G and Bielmann P (1981). Plasma vitamin A and precancerous lesions of cervix uteri: a preliminary report. Gynecol Oncology 11:136.

MacLennan R, Dalosta J, Day NE, Law CH, Ng YK and Shanmu-garatnam (1977). Risk factors for lung cancer in Singapore Chinese, a population with high female incidence rates. Int J Cancer 20:854.

Marshall J, Graham S, Mettlin C, Shedd D and Swanson M (1982). Diet in the epidemiology of oral cancer. Nutr Cancer 3: (in press).

Mettlin C and Graham S (1979). Dietary risk factors in human bladder cancer. Am J Epidemiol 110:255.

Mettlin C and Graham S (1979). Methodologic issues in etiologic studies of diet and colon cancer. Nutr Cancer 1:46.

Mettlin C, Graham S and Swanson M (1979). Vitamin A and lung cancer. J Natl Cancer Inst 62:1435.

Peto R, Doll R, Buckley JD and Sporn, MR (1981). Can dietary beta-carotene materially reduce human cancer rates? Nature 290:201.

Shekelle RB, Lepper M, Liu S, Maliza C, Raynor WJ, Jr, Rossof AH, Paul O, Shryock AM and Stamler J (1981). Dietary vitamin A and risk of cancer in the western electric study. Lancet 2:1185.

Wald N, Idle M, Boreham J and Bailey A (1980). Low serum-vitamin-A and subsequent risk of cancer. Lancet 2:813.

Wolbach SB and Howe PR (1925). Tissue changes following deprivation of fat-soluable A vitamin. J Exp Med 42:753.

MUTAGENS AND CANCER

Diet, Nutrition, and Cancer:
From Basic Research to Policy Implications, pages 137–139
© *1983 Alan R. Liss, Inc., 150 Fifth Avenue, New York, NY 10011*

NATURAL MUTAGENS: OVERVIEW

Joyce McCann, Ph.D.

Biomedical Division
Lawrence Berkeley Laboratory
University of California
Berkeley, California   94720

In the last 5-6 years, there have been literally thousands of chemicals, both man-made and natural, tested for
genotoxic activity. This has been brought about by the
development of rapid, relatively inexpensive genetic screening tests. There are now on the order of 100 of these tests
available that employ diverse organisms from bacteria and
mammalian cells in culture, to human cells. Some systems
even measure genotoxic effects in vivo in whole animals.
The rapid development of these systems was brought about
primarily as a consequence of the successful exploitation
of two important observations. First, the finding that
most chemical carcinogens are carcinogenic (or mutagenic)
only after metabolic conversion by enzyme systems in
mammalian tissues. This enabled the incorporation of
mammalian tissue extracts into simple in vitro systems.
Second, the increased understanding of the importance of
DNA repair in modulating effects of chemical carcinogens.
This permitted the development of very sensitive test
organisms capable of detection of a wide range of chemical
mutagens.

The application of genotoxic tests, the so-called short-
term tests, to man-made and natural chemicals has resulted
in the unexpected finding that there are many more mutagens,
especially natural mutagens, than we formerly thought. As
the speakers in this session will discuss, mutagens are
being discovered, at a still increasing rate, in many foods
that form an important part of our diet, such as cooked
meat, baked breads, and food vegetables. Mutagens are also
present in the water we drink and the air we breath; indeed

it appears that contact with mutagens is a daily event.

This new finding is challenging two important assumptions that have been made in chemical carcinogenesis. First,
the assumption that carcinogens are rare, and second, that
most carcinogens are man-made. The first assumption has
been fundamental both to theoretical considerations of the
mechanism of carcinogenesis, and to public policies aimed
at regulating human exposure to carcinogens. Somatic mutation theories of carcinogenesis that have focused on
initiation (mutagenesis) as the rate-limiting step (and
hence the most important to prevent) are clearly challenged
if the human mutagen burden is actually very large. After
all, even though the cancer rate is high, many people do
not get cancer. If the rate of initiation is much higher
than the cancer rate, it might imply that the later (promotional) stages in carcinogenesis are the more important
rate-limiting steps. In the policy area, policies (e.g.,
the Delaney Clause) have been risk averse, proposing that
identified carcinogens be banned, or human exposure
severely restricted.

Clearly, the impact of altering assumptions about the
prevalence of carcinogens would be enormous in both the
scientific and the policy areas. It is therefore critical
that we examine the validity of these new results with great
care. First, what is the relevance to humans of the tests
used to detect the mutagenic (and carcinogenic) activity
of these chemicals? Not only are there the obvious un-
certainties involved in extrapolating results obtained in
bacteria, or cells in culture, to a human being, but mutagenic activity, by it's very nature (at any particular
locus, it is a very rare event) requires high doses of mutagen for detection. We now know that some repair processes
that appear to be induced at high doses can result in mutagenesis. Thus, activity of mutagens in humans under environmental exposures, especially if they are much lower
than those used in mutagenesis tests, may be much less than
might be assumed by direct extrapolation of mutagenesis test
results.

Second, should there be any special significance
attached to whether a chemical is "natural" or "man-made"?
We do not know whether long exposure during evolution to
natural mutagens may have resulted in the development of
mechanisms aimed at protection against genotoxic effects of

those chemicals. Certainly some man-made chemicals, such as saccharin and some of the polychlorinated pesticides, have molecular structures that are new to our mammalian systems. Does this "foreign-ness" present a greater hazard?

Third, laboratory tests are traditionally carried out on pure chemicals, under isolated conditions, and yet humans are usually exposed to the same chemicals in complex mixtures. More and more chemicals are being discovered in the natural environment that can enhance or inhibit the genotoxic activity of other chemicals. How do complex mixtures modify the risk from exposure to genotoxic chemicals? For example, is it more hazardous to be ex-posed to nitrite in a protein-dense environment such as sausages, as compared to vegetables?

The finding that there are many natural mutagens is exciting in that it opens the way for new scientific approaches to understanding carcinogenesis. It is somewhat worrisome that it also provides a forceful argument against regulating man-made carcinogens for those whose interests are more economic or political than scientific. While we are in this period of fresh scientific discovery, where new observations are not yet in final perspective, and where their relevance to human cancer risk is far from certain, it is important that scientists continue to provide guidance that will insure that any changes in government regulatory policies are made cautiously, within the bounds of scientific reasonability.

Diet, Nutrition, and Cancer:
From Basic Research to Policy Implications, pages 141–154
© *1983 Alan R. Liss, Inc., 150 Fifth Avenue, New York, NY 10011*

THE IDENTIFICATION OF ANTIGENOTOXIC/ANTICARCINOGENIC AGENTS
IN FOOD

Miriam P. Rosin and Hans F. Stich

Environmental Carcinogenesis Unit
British Columbia Cancer Research Centre
601 West 10th Avenue
Vancouver, B.C., Canada V5Z 1L3

The last decade has seen the introduction of many sensitive, rapid and economic short-term assays for detecting
genotoxic agents in man's environment. A battery of these
tests is being widely used to assess the genetic and/or
carcinogenic hazard posed by chemicals to which man is
exposed. Less attention has been given to the design of
test systems to identify antigenotoxic and/or anticarcinogenic agents. Considering the important role now being
attributed to anticarcinogenic agents in controlling cancer
incidences, the existing gap of reliable bioassays should be
bridged as soon as possible. In this paper we discuss a few
of the more promising approaches for obtaining information on
the antigenotoxic/anticarcinogenic activities of food
products.

The Use of *In Vitro* Assays to Identify Antigenotoxic Agents

Short-term *in vitro* assays can be used to identify
compounds which suppress the genotoxic activity of carcinogens. This approach has already led to the identification
of numerous antigenotoxic agents among daily consumed food
components. Some of these naturally occurring inhibitors
are listed in Table 1.

The antigenotoxic agents of food products belong to
several chemical groups, e.g., vitamins, trace metals, fatty
acids and dietary fibers. These antigenotoxic agents are
consumed in fairly large quantities in our diet. For example, the plant phenolics are ubiquitously distributed in
fresh fruits and vegetables. Chlorogenic acid, caffeic acid

Table 1. Suppression of Genotoxicity by Food Components

Inhibitor	Genotoxic Agent	Reference
Ascorbate	Sterigmatocystin, DMN	1
	N-Nitrosoguanidine, DMN	2
	Malonaldehyde, β-propiolactone	3
	MNNG	4
Retinol	B(a)P	5
	OAAT	6
Retinol acetate	OAAT	6
Retinol palmitate	OAAT	6
α-Tocopherol	Malonaldehyde, β-propiolactone	3
Glutathione	N-Acetoxy-AAF	7
Cysteine	Hydroxylamine, hydrazine, isoniazid	8
	N-Acetoxy-AAF, N-hydroxy-AAF, MNNG, AFB_1, 4NQO, MMS, AF-2, nitrofurazone	9
Selenium	AAF, N-hydroxy-AAF	10
	Malonaldehyde, β-propiolactone	3
	B(a)P	5
	MNNG, N-acetoxy-AAF	4
Fe^{+++}, Fe^{++}	Cigarette smoke	11
Cu^{++}	Heated glucose-lysine	11
Oleic acid and Linoleic acid	Trp-P-1, Glu-P-1, Glob-P-2, IQ, B(a)P, AFB_1	12
Chlorophyllin	B(a)P	13
	Trp-P-1, Trp-P-2, Glu-P-1, Glu-P-2, amino-α-carboline, aminomethyl-α-carboline	14
Chlorogenic acid	MNNG, AFB_1	15
Caffeic acid	MNNG, AFB_1	15
Gallic acid	MNNG, AFB_1	15
Salicylic acid	AFB_1	15
p-Hydroxybenzoic acid	AFB_1	15
Coumaric acid	AFB_1	15
p-Cinnamic acid	AFB_1	15
Tannic acid	AFB_1	15
Catechol	AFB_1	15
Phenylethylisothio-cyanate	B(a)P	5
Phenylisothiocyanate	B(a)P	5

Table 1 (cont'd)

Inhibitor	Genotoxic Agent	Reference
Pectin	AFB_1, 2-NF	16
Lignin	AFB_1, 2-NF	16
Lambda carrageenan	AFB_1, 2-NF	16
Kappa carrageenan	AFB_1, 2-NF	16
Iota carrageenan	AFB_1, 2-NF	16
Cellulose	AFB_1, 2-NF	16
Corn bran	AFB_1	16
Maillard browning reaction products	AFB_1, MNNG	17
Caramelization products	AFB_1, MNNG	17
Vegetable and fruit juices	3-Methylcholanthrene, B(a)P	18,19,20
	Trp-P-1	21

Footnotes

References:

1: Lo and Stich (1978)
2: Guttenplan (1977)
3: Shamberger et al. (1979)
4: Rosin and Stich (1979)
5: Calle and Sullivan (1982)
6: Busk and Ahlorg (1982)
7: Rosin and Stich (1978a)
8: Speit et al. (1980)
9: Rosin and Stich (1978b)
10: Jacobs et al. (1977)
11: Rosin (1982)
12: Hayatsu et al. (1981)
13: Arimoto et al. (1980a)
14: Arimoto et al. (1980b)
15: Chan and Stich (manuscript in preparation)
16: Freeman et al. (manuscript in preparation)
17: Chan et al. (1982)
18: Lai et al. (1980)
19: Nishioka et al. (1981)
20: Tannenbaum et al. (1981)
21: Morita et al. (1978)

Abbreviations:

DMN, dimethylnitrosamine; MNNG, N-methyl-N'-nitro-N-nitrosoguanidine; B(a)P, benzo(a)pyrene; OAAT, ortho-aminoazotoluene; N-acetoxy-AAF, N-acetoxy-2-acetylaminofluorene; N-hydroxy-AAF, N-hydroxy-2-acetylaminofluorene; AFB_1, aflatoxin B_1; 4NQO, 4-nitroquinoline-1-oxide; MMS, methyl methanesulfonate; nitrofurazone, 5-nitro-2-furaldehyde semicarbazone; AF2, 2-(2-furyl)-3-(5-nitro-2-furyl)acrylamide; AAF, 2-acetylaminofluorene; Trp-P-1, 3-amino-1,4-dimethyl-5H-pyrido[4,3-b]-indole; Glu-P-1, 2-amino-6-methyl-dipyrido[1,2-a:3',2'-d]imidazole; Glob-P-2, 2-amino-9H-pyrido[2,3-b]indole; IQ, 2-amino-3-methylimidazo-[4,5-d]quinoline; Trp-P-2, 3-amino-1-methyl-5H-pyrido[4,3-b]indole; Glu-P-2, 2-amino-dipyrido[1,2-a:3',2'-d]imidazole; amino-α-carboline, 2-amino-9H-pyrido[2,3-b]indole; aminomethyl-α-carboline, 2-amino-3-methyl-9H-pyrido[2,3-b]indole; 2-NF, 2-nitrofluorene.

and gallic acid also occur in large quantities in regularly consumed beverages such as coffee and tea. One cup of coffee contains 250-260 mg chlorogenic acid. Approximately 64 mg of gallic acid has been found in 100 g of tea. It would thus appear that antigenotoxic components are readily available as natural components of food. The actual ingested quantities of such compounds varies considerably from individual to individual and between populations with different dietary patterns.

Antigenotoxic agents are not only indigenous to the foods we consume, but may be produced during the preparation of our food. The heating of sugar or sugar- and protein-containing foods to normal cooking temperatures (120-180°C) produces browning reaction products which possess a strong antigenotoxic activity (Chan *et al* 1982). For example, the Maillard reaction products formed during the heating of lysine and fructose (121°C, 1 hr) will suppress the mutagenic activity of the direct-acting carcinogen MNNG in cultures of *Salmonella typhimurium* TA1535. The same reaction products also inhibit the induction of reverse point mutations in *Salmonella* cultures exposed to aflatoxin B_1, an S9-requiring carcinogen (Fig. 1).

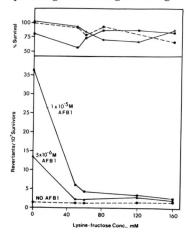 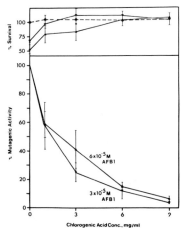

Fig. 1. Effect of heated lysine-fructose reaction products on cell survival and mutagenicity of AFB$_1$-treated *S. typhimurium* TA98.

Fig. 2. Suppression of AFB$_1$-induced mutagenicity by chlorogenic acid.

The advantages of *in vitro* short-term tests for genotoxicity and antigenotoxicity are their simplicity, speed and
economy. They can thus be used to screen large numbers of
chemicals or complex food mixtures within a reasonable timespan. There is one additional advantage to an *in vitro*
approach. Such studies can be used to obtain information on
the mechanism of action of antigenotoxic agents. For example,
the plant phenolic chlorogenic acid inhibits aflatoxin B_1-
induced mutagenicity in *Salmonella* cultures (Fig. 2). The
metabolites produced during a coincubation of aflatoxin B_1
and a liver S9 metabolizing system were separated with a high
pressure liquid chromatograph and examined with a fluorescent
detector (Fig. 3). Two new major peaks (5.8 and 6.1 min)
were generated due to metabolism of the aflatoxin B_1. When
chlorogenic acid was added to the reaction mixture, the formation of the aflatoxin B_1 metabolites was suppressed (Fig.
4). Chlorogenic acid would thus appear to affect the metabolism of the aflatoxin B_1 to mutagenic components.

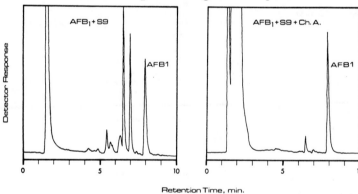

Fig. 3. HPLC profile of AFB_1
metabolites.

Fig. 4. HPLC profile when
chlorogenic acid (Ch.A.) is
present during AFB_1 activation
(R.I.M. Chan, M.Sc. Thesis).

Inhibitory Effect of Body Fluids

One limitation of the use of *in vitro* assays to identify
antigenotoxic food components is that such tests do not take
into account the vast array of biochemical alterations which
occur as food passes through the digestive tract. A kalei-
doscope of interactions will take place among the various
ingested food components as well as between these components

and the contents of the physiological fluids which surround them. Such changes may result in the suppression of the genotoxic activity of some chemicals while enhancing the activity of other components.

The *in vivo* events can be simulated "*in vitro*" by including various physiological fluids in short-term assays. This approach has led to the discovery of antigenotoxic activity in human saliva, gastric juice and serum (Table 2). Saliva seems to exert several types of protective effects against genotoxic agents. It can reduce the genotoxic activity of preformed carcinogens such as MNNG and it can suppress the endogenous formation of N-nitroso compounds.

Table 2. Inhibition of Genotoxicity or the Formation of Genotoxic Agents in Human Fluids

Sample Containing Inhibitors	Genotoxic Agents	Reference
Saliva	AF-2, MNNG, 4-NQO, AFB_1 B(a)P, Trp-P-1, quercetin, beef and salmon pyrolysates, cigarette smoke condensate	1
	Tannic acid	2
	Nitrosomethylurea formation	3
	N-Nitrosomorpholine formation	4
Gastric juice	Sodium dichromate, sodium azide	5
	N-Nitrosomorpholine formation	6
Serum	AF-2, 4NQO, B(a)P, quercetin	7

Footnotes

References:

1: Nishioka et al. (1981)
2: Stich et al. (1983b)
3: Stich et al. (1982)
4: Tannenbaum et al. (1978)
5: de Flora and Boido (1980)
6: Tannenbaum et al. (1981)
7: Nishioka (1983)

Abbreviations: see Table 1.

The close simulation of events which may occur during a meal is demonstrated with the following example. Salted fish was chosen due to its likely involvement in human cancers (Ho *et al* 1978). Nitrite-treated (pH 2, 1 hr, 37°C) fish extracts induce histidine revertants in strain TA1535 of *S. typhimurium* in the absence of an S9 activation mixture. The addition of human saliva to the nitrite/fish extract mixture at pH 2 reduces the formation of mutagenic reaction products (Fig. 5). Chinese or Indian tea also inhibit the formation of mutagenic nitrosation products. However, the inhibitory effects of saliva and tea are not additive under naturally occurring conditions.

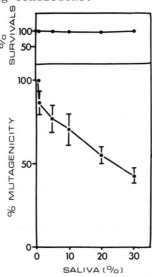

Fig. 5. The effect of human saliva on development of mutagenicity in nitrite-treated salted fish.

These results point to a possible involvement of saliva in chemical carcinogenesis. Nishioka *et al* (1981) have shown that human saliva can inactivate the mutagenic activity of a wide spectrum of carcinogens, including those formed during cooking (Table 2). We have observed a similar ability of saliva to reduce the clastogenic activity of several compounds which are ingested daily in mg quantities (Table 3).

Whether or not these results are indicative of the *in vivo* situation is not yet known. However, the incidence of tumors is reduced in rats following the joint application of 4-nitroquinoline-1-oxide (4NQO) and 7,12-dimethylbenz(a)-

Table 3. Effect of Human Saliva on Clastogenic Activity of Naturally Occurring Genotoxic Compounds (CHO cells were exposed to the phenolics for 3 hrs)

Chemical	Concentration (mg/ml)	% Metaphases with Chromosome Aberrations	
		Alone	+Saliva*
Tannic acid	0.1	51.4	3.0
Gallic acid	0.012	25.9	1.3
Caffeic acid	0.25	10.0	0.0
Chlorogenic acid	1.0	22.2	0.0

*1 part saliva:3 parts culture medium.

anthracene (DMBA) and saliva (Wallenius 1966) and an increased tumor frequency following an inhibition of salivary secretion (Wallenius, Lekholm 1973).

The possible ramifications of this protective role of saliva are intriguing. It has been suggested that genotoxic effects in target cells in the mouth may only result when the concentration of genotoxic agents in the saliva exceeds the level which can be inhibited by the saliva (Stich *et al* 1983a). Such a situation may be occurring among betel nut and tobacco chewers. The release of genotoxic agents into the saliva of these chewers has been linked to the development of cancers in the exposed target tissues. Individuals who spit during their chewing period develop cancers of the oral cavity and pharynx. Swallowing of the saliva during chewing is associated with the development of esophageal cancers. Future studies involving the identification of the inhibitory components in the saliva, the quantification of these components in various individuals, and the elucidation of environmental (e.g., dietary) and genetic controls for these components may help our understanding of protection mechanisms which can operate before the genome of cells is altered.

Development of Tests for Human Population Groups

The *in vitro* approaches are efficient methods for screening our environment for modulators of carcinogen activity. However, the extrapolation of *in vitro* results to man has always been a matter of concern. It is, of course, possible to further examine the more promising "antigeno-toxic" agents for an anticarcinogenic activity in animals. The advantage of this approach lies in the ability to copy more closely exposure patterns to which man may be submitted (Wattenberg 1979). Anticarcinogens can be applied prior to, during or after exposure to carcinogens. However, the extent to which results obtained on inbred mice can be used to predict a response in a genetically heterogenous human population group still remains an unresolved issue.

The role of anticarcinogens in human cancer incidences is primarily suggested by results from epidemiological analyses of various high and low risk population groups. For example, the regular consumption of green and yellow vegetables has been associated with decreased cancer frequencies (Hirayama 1982). In another instance, the lack of fresh fruits and vegetables in the Linxian county of China has been linked to an increased incidence of cancer of the esophagus, an occurrence felt to be related to the paucity of blocking agents for nitrosamine formation (Yang 1980). It is not yet known whether epidemiological methods have the resolving power to unravel the multitude of dietary factors which can suppress or enhance carcinogenicity. An answer to this dilemma may reside in the development of more "*in vivo*" genotoxicity tests which are directly applicable to population groups consuming what may be called "low risk" and "high risk" diets.

We have focused our attention on the possible use of micronuclei formation in exfoliated human cells as a method of estimating the efficiency of anticarcinogenic agents. As a first step in this endeavour, we examined buccal mucosa cells of individuals at high risk for oral cancers: (a) raw betel nut eaters (Khasis of the northeastern hills of India), (b) betel quid (pan) chewers in India, (c) tobacco chewers (Khaini chewers of India), and (d) heavy smokers (two packs or more per day) and alcohol drinkers in British Columbia. A preliminary study of Indian betel quid and tobacco chewers was recently completed (Stich *et al* 1983c,d). In each case, an elevated frequency of micronucleated buccal mucosa cells was found. Five of the examined local smokers and drinkers also had an increased frequency of micronucleated mucosa cells over that found in a non-smoking, non-drinking population group. The one exception proved, upon rechecking, to be a health-conscious person taking 2 g of ascorbate and vitamin A per day. We have currently extended our studies of micronuclei frequencies to exfoliated cells of the respiratory tract and the urine. Their "background" frequencies vary between 0.0 and 1%. Thus the action of carcinogens should be readily detectable by an increase in their frequencies.

The temporal pattern of formation of micronucleated exfoliated cells in response to a carcinogen has been studied by examining buccal mucosa cells from cancer patients receiving radiotherapy to the head and neck region. These individuals receive radiation treatments Monday through Friday for a duration of 4 to 6 weeks. The frequency of micronucleated mucosa cells from the irradiated area increased throughout the course of therapy (Fig. 6). Once the radiation exposure is terminated, the clastogenic effect ceases and the micronucleated cells in the mucosa start to disappear (Fig. 7).

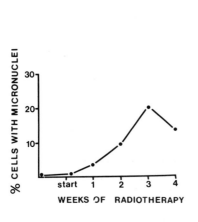

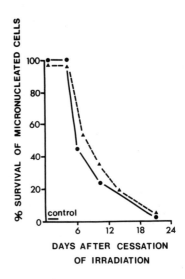

Fig. 6. Development of micronuclei in buccal mucosa cells during radiotherapy to the cheek. Patient (38 years old) received a total of 4744 rads during the 4-week period.

Fig. 7. Disappearance of micronuclei after cessation of radiotherapy in two patients who received a total of 3000 and 6000 rads, respectively to the buccal mucosa.

The above-described behaviour of micronucleated cells during the after exposure to carcinogenic agents suggests an approach that can be taken to estimate the efficiency of intervention (chemoprevention) programs. We would like to exemplify such a pattern on betel quid or chewing tobacco users, since a considerable amount of background information is already available (Fig. 8). A relatively high frequency

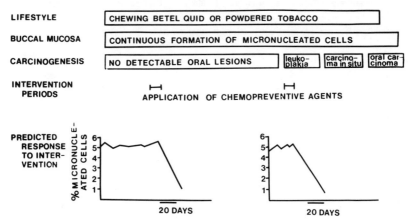

Fig. 8. Micronucleated exfoliated cells as a tool to assess intervention.

of micronucleated cells can be found in the mucosa of chewers long before any preneoplastic lesions are detectable. The cessation of chewing or a successful intervention program should be reflected in a reduction of micronucleated mucosa cells. This response should become obvious within about 14 to 21 days after prevention treatment has occurred. In our opinion, it requires only one or two cell generation times plus the migration time from the basal cell layer to the surface to see a significant reduction of micronucleated cells. The actual timespan may be shorter than one would expect from the radiation studies shown in Fig. 7 because of the large doses administered during therapy which may delay the cell cycle.

To judge the usefulness of the proposed approach, one must keep in mind that the frequency of micronucleated exfoliated cells does not reflect a particular stage in carcinogenesis but only provides evidence of exposure to clastogenic chemical or physical carcinogens. Although the proposed protocol is based on our experience with the buccal mucosa of betel nut, betel quid or powdered tobacco chewers, the principle can be readily applied to high risk population groups for esophageal cancers (exfoliated cells obtainable by the balloon or brush procedure), nasopharyngeal carcinomas (cells obtainable by swab procedure) or urinary bladder cancers (cells obtainable from the urine). In these and other cases, the frequency of micronuclei can be used as an internal dosimeter to monitor exposure patterns to carcinogens in the tissue from which tumors will arise.

Acknowledgements

These studies were supported by the Strategic Grants Program of the Natural Sciences and Engineering Research Council of Canada and by the National Cancer Institute of Canada.

References

Arimoto S, Negishi T, Hayatsu H (1980a). Inhibitory effect of hemin on the mutagenic activities of carcinogens. Cancer Lett 11:29.

Arimoto S, Ohara Y, Namba T, Negishi T, Hayatsu H (1980b). Inhibition of the mutagenicity of amino acid pyrolysis products by hemin and other biological pyrrole pigments. Biochem Biophys Res Commun 92:662.

Busk L, Ahlorg UG (1982). Retinoids as inhibitors of ortho-aminoazotoluene-induced mutagenesis in the Salmonella/ liver microsome test. Mutat Res 104:225.

Calle LM, Sullivan PD (1982). Screening of antioxidants and other compounds for antimutagenic properties towards benzo-(a)pyrene-induced mutagenicity in strain TA98 of *Salmonella typhimurium*. Mutat Res 101:99.

Chan RIM, Stich HF, Rosin MP, Powrie WD (1982). Antimuta-genic activity of browning reaction products. Cancer Lett 15:27.

de Flora S, Boido V (1980). Effect of human gastric juice on the mutagenicity of chemicals. Mutat Res 77:307.

Guttenplan JB (1977). Inhibition by L-ascorbate of bacterial mutagenesis induced by two N-nitroso compounds. Nature (Lond) 268:368.

Hayatsu H, Arimoto S, Togawa K, Makita M (1981). Inhibitory effect of the ether extract of human feces on activities of mutagens: inhibition by oleic and linoleic acids. Mutat Res 81:287.

Hirayama T (1982). Epidemiology of human carcinogenesis: a review of food-related diseases. In Stich HF (ed): "Carcinogens and Mutagens in the Environment", Vol I, "Food Products", Boca Raton, Florida: CRC Press, in press.

Ho JHC, Huang DP, Fong YY (1978). Salted fish and nasopharyngeal carcinoma in southern China. Lancet ii:626.

Jacobs MM, Matney TS, Griffin CA (1977). Inhibitory effects of selenium on the mutagenicity of 2-acetylaminofluorene (AAF) and AAF derivatives. Cancer Lett 2:319.

Lai C-N, Butler MA, Matney TS (1980). Antimutagenic activities of common vegetables and their chlorophyll content. Mutat Res 77:245.

Lo LW, Stich HF (1978). The use of short-term tests to measure the preventive action of reducing agents on formation and activation of carcinogenic nitroso compounds. Mutat Res 57:57.

Morita K, Hara M, Kada T (1978). Studies on natural desmutagens: screening for vegetable and fruit factors active in inactivation of mutagenic pyrolysis products of amino acids. Agric Biol Chem 42:1235.

Nishioka H (1983). Antimutagenic activity of human saliva and serum. In Stich HF (ed): "Carcinogens and Mutagens in the Environment", Vol II, "Naturally Occurring Compounds", Boca Raton, Florida: CRC Press, in press.

Nishioka H, Nishi K, Kyokane K (1981). Human saliva inactivates mutagenicity of carcinogens. Mutat Res 85:323.

Rosin MP (1982). Inhibition of genotoxic activities of complex mixtures by naturally occurring agents. In Stich HF (ed): "Carcinogens and Mutagens in the Environment", Vol I, "Food Products", Boca Raton, Florida: CRC Press, in press.

Rosin MP, Stich HF (1978a). The inhibitory effect of reducing agents on N-acetoxy- and N-hydroxy-2-acetylaminofluorene-induced mutagenesis. Cancer Res 38:1307.

Rosin MP, Stich HF (1978b). The inhibitory effect of cysteine on the mutagenic activities of several carcinogens. Mutat Res 54:73.

Rosin MP, Stich HF (1979). Assessment of the use of the Salmonella mutagenesis assay to determine the influence of antioxidants on carcinogen-induced mutagenesis. Int J Cancer 23:722.

Shamberger RJ, Corlett CL, Beaman KD, Kasten BL (1979). Antioxidants reduce the mutagenic effect of malonaldehyde and β-propiolactone. Part IX. Antioxidants and cancer. Mutat Res 66:349.

Speit G, Wick C, Wolf M (1980). Induction of sister chromatid exchanges by hydroxylamine, hydrazine and isoniazid and their inhibition by cysteine. Human Genet 54:155.

Stich HF, Rosin MP, Bryson L (1982). The inhibitory effect of whole and deproteinized saliva on mutagenicity and clastogenicity resulting from a model nitrosation reaction. Mutat Res, in press.

Stich HF, Bohm B, Chatterjee K, Sailo J (1983a). The role of saliva-borne mutagens and carcinogens in the etiology of oral and esophageal carcinomas of betel nut and tobacco chewers. In Stich HF (ed): "Carcinogens and Mutagens in the Environment", Vol II, "Naturally Occurring Compounds", Boca Raton, Florida: CRC Press, in press.

Stich HF, Chan PKL, Rosin MP (1983b). Inhibitory effects of naturally occurring phenolics and saliva on the formation of mutagenic nitrosation products of salted fish. Int J Cancer, in press.

Stich HF, Stich W, Parida BB (1983c). Elevated frequency of micronucleated cells in the buccal mucosa of individuals at high risk for oral cancer: betel quid chewers. Cancer Lett, in press.

Stich HF, Curtis R, Parida BB (1983d). Application of the micronucleus test to exfoliated cells of high cancer risk groups: tobacco chewers. Int J Cancer, in press.

Tannenbaum SR, Archer MC, Wishnok JS, Bishop WW (1978). Nitrosamine formation in human saliva. J Natl Cancer Inst 60:251.

Tannenbaum SR, Moran D, Falchuk KR, Correa P, Cuello C (1981). Nitrite stability and nitrosation potential in human gastric juice. Cancer Lett 14:131.

Wallenius K (1966). Experimental oral cancer in the rat, with special reference to the influence of saliva. Acta path microbiol scand 180, Suppl:1.

Wallenius K, Lekholm V (1973). Influence of saliva on epidermal cancer in rats induced by water- or fat-soluble carcinogens. Odont Revy 24:115.

Wattenberg LW (1979). Naturally occurring inhibitors of chemical carcinogenesis. In Miller EC, Miller JA, Hirono I, Sugimura T, Takayama S (eds): "Naturally Occurring Carcinogens-Mutagens and Modulators of Carcinogenesis", Tokyo: Jap Sci Soc Press/Baltimore: Univ Park Press, p 315.

Yang CS (1980). Research on esophageal cancer in China: a review. Cancer Res 40:2633.

Diet, Nutrition, and Cancer:
From Basic Research to Policy Implications, pages 155–165
© *1983 Alan R. Liss, Inc., 150 Fifth Avenue, New York, NY 10011*

MYCOTOXIN CONTRIBUTION TO THE HUMAN MUTAGEN BURDEN

D.P.H. Hsieh, M. Fukayama, D.W. Rice

Department of Environmental Toxicology
University of California, Davis, CA 95616

FOOD SAFETY SIGNIFICANCE OF MYCOTOXINS

Mycotoxins are toxic metabolites produced by fungi that develop in food crops and food commodities. Their widespread occurrence under a broad range of environmental conditions makes them a major source of natural toxins in foods (Ciegler, Burmeister, Vesonder, Hesseltine 1981). Ingestion of mycotoxins through contaminated foodstuffs by humans at parts per billion (ppb) levels is practically unavoidable. Even at these low levels, certain mycotoxins present a considerable hazard due to their potent mutagenicity and carcinogenicity. For example, aflatoxin B_1 (AFB_1), a mycotoxin produced by <u>Aspergillus flavus</u>, is the most potent hepatocarcinogen ever known. In a recent ranking of carcinogens for regulatory priorities, AFB_1 was recognized as the one posing the highest potential risk to humans (Squire 1981).

Due to the extremely high carcinogenicity of AFB_1 and its frequent presence in peanuts, corn, cottonseed and other foodstuffs, there has been a great concern that mycotoxins may be a significant class of naturally occurring carcinogens in food. This legitimate concern has been an impetus in the worldwide active investigation of mycotoxins in the last twenty years.

For a mycotoxin to be considered significant in human food safety, it must meet at least three criteria: it must be highly toxic to bioassay systems, it must be present at significant levels in food commodities, and it must be

involved in the etiology of certain specific human and
animal diseases. The major mycotoxins currently viewed as
significant from a regulation standpoint are mostly produced
by three genera of fungi: Aspergillus, Penicillium, and
Fusarium.

MUTAGENIC MYCOTOXINS AND THEIR CARCINOGENICITY

Recent advancement in genetic toxicology has made
available a number of short-term genotoxicity tests that are
useful in detecting the potential capability of mycotoxins
to initiate carcinogenesis in animals (Stark 1980). The
most frequently used are three microbial mutagenicity tests:
the reverse mutation test using histidine auxotrophs of the
bacterium Salmonella typhimurium (Ames, McCann, Yamasaki
1975; Ueno, Kubota, Ito, Nakamura 1978; Wehner, Thiel, Van
Rensberg, Demasius 1978), the growth inhibition (rec effect)
test using the recombination deficient mutant of the bacterium Bacillus subtilis (Ueno, Kubota 1976), and the forward
mutation test using the yeast Saccharomyces cerevisiae
(Kuczuk, Benson, Heath, Hayes 1978). The mutagenicity of
some significant mycotoxins as detected by these three
microbial tests and the carcinogenicity of these mycotoxins
are compared in Table 1. A positive result to any of the
three mutagenicity tests is considered positive (+) in
mutagenicity; the ability to induce tumors in any species of
animals regardless of routes of administration is considered
positive (+) in carcinogenicity. The comparison indicates
that the three microbial mutagenicity tests as a battery
give two false positives (PR toxin and rubratoxin B) and one
false negative (T-2 toxin) of the 14 mycotoxins compared.

A shortcoming of the microbial mutagenicity tests is
their inability to detect epigenetic carcinogens which exert
their effects through promotion, rather than initiation.
Also, the microbial test systems are artificially sensitized
single cells that provide genetic targets for a test chemical to express the ensuing genetic damage in the form of a
specific mutation. They do not contain the complex biological barriers found in animals which determine the
metabolic fate of a test chemical and its bioavailability at
the genetic target sites. Due to the artificially minimized
biological barriers remaining in the microbial test systems,
the susceptibility of these systems to the chemical is
considerably higher than the target animal cells in vivo.

Table 1. The Mutagenicity and Carcinogenicity of Mycotoxins

Mycotoxin	Carcinogenicity	Mutagenicity
Aspergillus toxins		
Aflatoxin B_1	+	+
Aflatoxin G_1	+	+
Aflatoxin M_1	+	+
Sterigmatocystin	+	+
Ochratoxin A	−	−
Penicillium toxins		
Citrinin	+	+
Patulin	+	+
Penicillic acid	+	+
PR toxin	−	+
Rubratoxin B	−	+
Fusarium toxins		
Fusarenon X	nt	+
Nevalenol	nt	+
T-2 toxin	+	−
Zearalenone	+	+

nt = not tested; data derived from Stark (1980)

So far, AFB_1 is the only mycotoxin found to be carcinogenic to all the animal species used in testing. Aflatoxins are also the only class of mycotoxins that has received adequate epidemiological studies and has been found to be associated with an increased cancer risk in certain human populations (Carlborg 1979). Similar epidemiological studies are unlikely to be conducted for other carcinogenic mycotoxins because of the cost and the complexity of epidemiological studies.

MUTAGEN BURDEN CONCEPT

The cost and difficulties of epidemiological studies and the shortcomings of currently available short-term mutagenicity tests have prompted the recent development of a mutagen burden concept to attempt a better tool for estimating and predicting the carcinogenic potential of major classes of environmental mutagens, including mycotoxins. This concept, initially advanced by a National Cancer Institute Task Force headed by Alexander Hollaender, takes into consideration the somatic mutation theory of carcinogenesis which underlies the correlation between the mutagenicity of a chemical and its ability to initiate carcinogenesis and the bioavailability of the chemical which determines how much of the chemical would reach the genetic target sites to cause somatic mutation. Operationally, the mutagen burden due to a chemical can be defined as the quantity of effective lesions in DNA caused by a chemical in an exposed human or animal. This definition implies that mutagenic and carcinogenic events induced by a chemical are proportional to the effective lesions in DNA caused by the chemical. Thus the mutagen burden due to a chemical is a function of the following three independent variables:

1. Level of exposure to the chemical in the environment.

2. Bioavailability of the active form of the chemical at the target DNA.

3. Capability of the chemical to cause effective lesions in DNA.

The exposure level of a chemical in the environment, in ng per kg body weight (BW) per day, can be determined by multiplying the concentrations of the chemical (e.g. µg of AFB_1 per kg diet) in various environmental media (e.g. air, water, food) with the daily intake of the appropriate media (e.g. kg diet per person per day) and then divided by the average BW per person.

The bioavailability of the active form of a chemical at target DNA can be assumed to be proportional to the amount of chemical bound to DNA such as the in vivo "Covalent Binding Index" (CBI), that was defined by Lutz (1979):

$$CBI = \frac{\text{damage to DNA}}{\text{dose}}$$

$$= \frac{\text{micromole chemical bound per mole nucleotides}}{\text{millimole chemical administered per kg animal}}$$

The capability of a chemical at the target site to cause effective lesions in DNA is reflected by the mutagenic potency of the chemical in a mutagenicity test such as the Ames Salmonella/microsome mutagenicity test. The end-point scored in such a mutagenicity test can be viewed as a biological expression of the effective DNA lesions that have escaped DNA-repair.

Thus the mutagen burden (MB) due to a chemical can be expressed as the product of the exposure level (D), the CBI, and the mutagenic potency (MP) of the chemical:

$$MB = D \times CBI \times MP$$

It is important to note that MB values are meaningful only in comparing the relative sigificance of two mutagens, therefore the CBI and MP values used in calculation should be those relative to a selected reference mutagen.

To evaluate the relative mutagenic potency of a chemical, a mutagen of established human carcinogenicity can be chosen as a reference mutagen for comparison, using a selected mutagenicity test operated under the appropriate optimal conditions for each chemical. For example, the Ames test can be a mutagenicity test of choice because of its general acceptance and the demonstrated correlation between the carcinogenicity and the mutagenicity of a large number of chemicals detected by this test, especially aflatoxins (McCann, Choi, Yamasaki, Ames 1975; Wong, Hsieh 1976). In view of its high potency as a carcinogen and mutagen and its demonstrated human carcinogenicity, AFB_1 can be a model reference mutagen of choice.

MUTAGEN BURDEN AND RELATIVE CARCINOGENIC POTENCY

Comparison of the potencies of some known carcinogens by Bruce Ames and his associates at the University of California (Maugh 1978) has revealed that there are orders of magnitude differences in the potencies among these carcinogens. The potency is expressed as the daily dose of a carcinogen in µg/kg BW/day that is required to induce tumors in 50% of a group of rats or mice over the course of their lifetimes. There is an eight-hundred-fold difference in potency between AFB_1 and dimethylnitrosamine and a two-million-fold difference between AFB_1 and saccharin. It is obvious that the mutagen burden of a person resulting from exposure to dimethylnitrosamine or to saccharin is negligible if he is also exposed to AFB_1 at similar levels. Similarly, the human mutagen burden contributed by AFB_1 may represent a large portion of the burden contributed by the entirety of mycotoxins.

Recently, much concern was aroused over aflatoxin M_1 (AFM_1), a hydroxylated metabolite of AFB_1 frequently detected in commercial milk and other dairy products (Stoloff 1980). This concern is based on the observation that AFM_1 and AFB_1 have similar acute toxicities in a number of bioassay systems and that AFM_1 is about 3% as mutagenic as AFB_1 in the Ames test (Wong, Hsieh 1976). Other short-term tests also indicate that AFM_1 is definitely genotoxic (Lutz 1979; Green, Rice, Hsieh, Byard 1982). An evaluation of MB, however, has revealed that AFM_1 is at least 200 times less carcinogenic than AFB_1 as shown in the following calculations.

The CBI's of AFB_1 and AFM_1 in the rat were determined by Lutz (1979) to be 10300 and 1600 respectively. The mutagenic potency of AFM_1 in the Ames test is 3% that of AFB_1. In a controlled experiment, if rats are given the same dose of AFB_1 or AFM_1, the carcinogenicity of AFM_1 as relative to that of AFB_1 in the rat can be estimated by comparing the MB due to the two toxins:

$$\frac{MB(B_1)}{MB(M_1)} = \frac{D(10300)(1)}{D(1600)(0.03)} = \frac{215}{1}$$

Using MB as an index of carcinogenicity, the potency of AFM_1 in the rat is therefore predicted to be less than 1/200 that of AFB_1, rather than 3% as predicted by the mutagenicity of AFM_1 alone. The carcinogenic potency of AFM_1 so predicted is in line with the result of a chronic study we have recently completed. In this study, male Fischer rats, a sensitive model, were continuously fed a diet containing 50 ppb of AFB_1 or AFM_1, a level 100 times greater than the action level of AFM_1 in milk. At the end of 18 months, multi-hepatocarcinomas were found in 100% of the AFB_1 group whereas no evidence of neoplasm was found in any of the AFM_1 group.

RISK ASSESSMENT

To compare the human cancer risk due to AFB_1 and AFM_1 in the United States the exposure levels of the two toxins need to be taken into consideration. Surveillance of occurrence of AFB_1 in foodstuffs has revealed that the principal sources of AFB_1 are peanut products and corn (Stoloff 1977). The average concentrations of AFB_1 in peanut products (PP) and in corn are 0.19 and 0.02 µg/kg respectively. These values are obtained by multiplication of the average concentrations of all samples analyzed (in µg/kg) and the incidence of contamination (in %). The average per capita consumption rates of these commodities from 1960 through 1980 are 7.6 g PP and 135 g corn per person per day (USDA 1981a). Assuming that the average body weight of a person is 50 kg, the daily intake of AFB_1 (DB) from diet can be calculated as

$$DB = \frac{(0.19 \text{ µg } AFB_1/\text{kg PP})(7.6 \text{ g PP/person/day})}{50 \text{ kg BW/person}} +$$

$$\frac{(0.02 \text{ µg } AFB_1/\text{kg corn})(135 \text{ g corn/person/day})}{50 \text{ kg BW/person}}$$

$$= 0.08 \text{ ng/kg BW/day}$$

Human exposure to AFM_1 is mainly through ingestion of contaminated dairy products (Stoloff 1980). The average per capita consumption rate of dairy products from 1960 through 1980 is calculated to be equivalent to 242 g of milk per person per day (USDA 1981b). The action level for AFM_1 in milk currently enforced by the Food and Drug Administration is 0.5 µg/kg. Assuming that the average concentration of AFM_1 in commercial milk is one-half of the action level, namely 0.25 µg/kg, the average daily intake of AFM_1(DM) is therefore

$$DM = \frac{0.25 \ \mu g/kg \ milk)(242 \ g \ milk/person/day)}{50 \ kg \ BW/person}$$

$$= 1.21 \ ng/kg \ BW/day$$

Assuming that the ratio of CBI of AFB_1 and AFM_1 in the human is similar to the ratio in the rat, the relative cancer risk from the two toxins as estimated by their respective contribution to the human MB is

$$\frac{MB \ (AFB_1)}{MB \ (AFM_1)} = \frac{219 \ (0.08)}{1 \ (1.21)} = 14$$

Thus the human cancer risk due to exposure to AFB_1 is, on average, about 14 times greater than that due to exposure to AFM_1, as predicted by the mutagen burden concept.

EVALUATION

The mutagen burden concept offers a way to utilize the mutagenicity data and the bioavailability data of a chemical to quantitatively predict the relative carcinogenic potency of a chemical. Therefore the predictive accuracy is better than using the mutagenicity alone. The inclusion of bio-availability in the evaluation of the mutagen burden allows the effects of dietary factors to be reflected in the prediction of the carcinogenicity of a chemical. This is because many dietary factors are known to modulate the car-cinogenicity of a chemical largely through their alterations of the bioavailability of the chemical (Wattenberg 1980). The use of CBI of a chemical, in particular, allows the organ specificity, the route of administration, and the selection of an animal model to be reflected in the evalua-tion of the bioavailability of the chemical.

In the evaluation of human MB contributed by AFB_1 and AFM_1, the following assumptions were made:

1. The mutagenicity of a chemical as measured by a selected mutagenicity test is accurately reflecting the effective lesions in the DNA to cause somatic mutation.

2. The ratio of the CBI's of two carcinogens compared in humans is similar to that in the rat or in any other selected animal model for the CBI determination.

3. There is a homogeneous occurrence of mycotoxins in food commodities; the per capita daily intake of contaminated foodstuffs is constant; the average BW of a person is 50 kg.

Obviously some of the assumptions are very crude. They can be refined by using data obtained from better designed experiments to improve the predictive value of the mutagen burden of a chemical.

SUMMARY

Mycotoxins are a significant class of naturally occurring carcinogens in food. The human mutagen burden contributed by mycotoxins may be represented by that contributed by aflatoxins because of their extremely high potency. Mutagen burden takes into consideration the bioavailability of a chemical and its mutagenicity in predicting the relative carcinogenic potency of the chemical. Its predictive value is better than that of mutagenicity alone. Inclusion of bioavailability in the evaluation of mutagen burden allows the effect of dietary factors on the carcinogenicity of a chemical to be reflected in the prediction. Mutagen burdens contributed by AFM_1 and by AFB_1 indicate that AFM_1 is at least 200 times less carcinogenic than AFB_1 in the adult rat at the same dose levels and that the potential human carcinogenic hazard posed by AFM_1 is 1/14 that of AFB_1.

ACKNOWLEDGMENT

The authors' research in this subject is supported in part by USPHS grants CA 27246 and ES 07059, National Dairy Council, Western Regional Research Project W-122, and Stauffer Chemical Company Fellowship.

REFERENCES

Ames BN, McCann J, Yamasaki E (1975). Methods for detecting carcinogens and mutagens with the Salmonella/mammalian-microsome mutagenicity test. Mutat Res 31:347.
Carlborg FW (1979). Cancer, mathematical models and aflatoxin. Fd Cosmet Toxicol 17:159.

Ciegler A, Burmeister HR, Vesonder RF, Hesseltine CW (1981). Mycotoxins: Occurrence in the environment. In Shank RC (ed.): "Mycotoxins and N-Nitroso Compounds: Environmental Risks. Vol I," Boca Raton, FL: CRC Press, p 1.

Green CE, Rice DW, Hsieh DPH, Byard JL (1982). The comparative metabolism and toxic potency of aflatoxin B_1 and aflatoxin M_1 in primary cultures of adult-rat hepatocytes. Toxicol Appl Pharmacol 20:53.

Kuczuk MH, Benson PM, Heath H, Hayes AW (1978). Evaluation of the mutagenic potential of mycotoxins using Salmonella typhimurium and Saccharomyces cerevisiae. Mutat Res 53:11.

Lutz WK (1979). In vivo covalent binding of organic chemicals to DNA as a quantitative indicator in the process of chemical carcinogenesis. Mutat Res 65:289.

Maugh TH (1978). Estimating potency of carcinogens is an inexact science. Science 202:38.

McCann J, Choi E, Yamasaki E, Ames BN (1975). Detection of carcinogens as mutagens in the Salmonella/microsome test: Assay of 300 chemicals. Proc Natl Acad Sci, USA 72:5135.

Squire RA (1981). Ranking animal carcinogens: A proposed regulatory approach. Science 214:877.

Stark A-A (1980). Mutagenicity and carcinogenicity of mycotoxins: DNA binding as a possible mode of action. Ann Rev Microbiol 34:235.

Stoloff L (1977). Aflatoxins--An overview. In Rodricks JV, Hesseltine CW, Mehlman MA (eds): "Mycotoxins: In Human and Animal Health," Illinois: Pathotox, p 7.

Stoloff L (1980). Aflatoxin M_1 in perspective. J Food Prot 43:226.

Ueno Y, Kubota K (1976). DNA-attacking ability of carcinogenic mycotoxins in recombination-deficient mutant cells of Bacillus subtilus. Cancer Res 35:382.

Ueno Y, Kubota K, Ito T, Nakamura Y (1978). Mutagenicity of carcinogenic mycotoxins in Salmonella typhimurium. Cancer Res 38:536.

USDA (1981a). Food consumption, prices and expenditures, 1960-1980. In Economic Research Service, Statistical Bulletin, No 672, p 62 and p 75.

USDA (1981b). Food consumption, prices and expenditures, 1960-1980. In Economic Research Service, Statistical Bulletin, No 672, p 9.

Wattenberg LW (1980). Inhibitors of chemical carcinogens. J Environ Pathol Toxicol 3:35.

Wehner FC, Thiel PG, Van Rensburg SJ, Demasius IPC (1978). Mutagenicity to Salmonella typhimurium of some Fusarium mycotoxins. Appl Environ Microbiol 35:659.

Wong JJ, Hsieh DPH (1976). Mutagenicity of aflatoxins related to their metabolism and carcinogenic potential. Proc Natl Acad Sci 73:2241.

Diet, Nutrition, and Cancer:
From Basic Research to Policy Implications, pages 167–176
© *1983 Alan R. Liss, Inc., 150 Fifth Avenue, New York, NY 10011*

PROTEASE INHIBITORS IN THE DIET AS ANTICARCINOGENS

Walter Troll and Jonathan Yavelow

New York University Medical Center
550 First Avenue
New York, NY 10016

Protease Inhibitors as Anticarcinogens

Protease inhibitors occur in multiple forms in many tissues throughout the entire plant and animal world, as well as in microorganisms. Although their role in biology and nutrition is not understood fully, their main physiological function seems to be to prevent proteolysis which could result in injury. In this capacity, they are valuable tools to study the role of proteolysis in carcinogenesis as well as in a number of biological disorders, such as inflammation and emphysema. They also have become of great interest nutritionally because of their high concentration in many seeds and storage organs of plants.

Their presence in the seeds and leaves of some plants suggests that they may be used as protective agents against insect infestation by inhibiting insect proteases. It first was observed that the larvae of certain insects were unable to develop normally on soybean products. Since this observation was made, Ryan has shown that insect wounding of a single leaf of a tomato or potato plant causes the accumulation of a protease inhibitor throughout the entire plant. This protective device can be considered to be a primitive immune system used by plants to protect themselves against invasion by insects (1). In man, protease inhibitors play a role in controlling disease. The α_1-trypsin inhibitor, which is present in our blood, prevents emphysema. The inhibitor can also be destroyed in individuals who are heavy smokers (2-4). Cigarette smoke contains particles which activate polymorphonuclear leukocytes or macrophages resulting in the formation of superoxide anions ($O_2^-\cdot$) and hydrogen peroxide (H_2O_2). The latter compound reacting with myeloperoxidase oxidizes the methionine in the prosthetic group of α_1-trypsin inhibitor, thus destroying its activity (5). Inactivation of the trypsin inhibitor, observed in cigarette smokers with emphysema, could also be a necessary condition of lung cancer.

Protease inhibitors also prevent mutations in micro-organisms. They prevent mutations in E. coli by preventing hydrolysis of genetic protein repressors (6). Mutations in bacteria have been a successful method of identifying geno-toxic agents in our environment.

Epidemiological studies have pointed to diet as a factor in cancer occurrence in man. The incidence of breast, colon and other cancers is lower in populations eating vegetarian diets. In particular, Seventh-Day Adventists, a vegetarian population, have a lower incidence of cancer than the general population (7). A lower incidence of breast, colon and prostatic cancers has also been correlated with high legume and cereal consumption (8,9). The occurrence of breast and colon cancers throughout the world is directly proportional to meat and fat consumption (10). Thus, it appears that not only may cancer incidence decrease if less fat (meat) is consumed; but that diets rich in legumes may contain protective factors, among them protease inhibitors, which may protect against many human cancers.

Carcinogenesis--a Multistage Process

The existence of at least two distinct phases in chemical carcinogenesis, termed initiation and promotion, is now well established (11,12). The initiator is a physical or a chemical agent applied in a single subcarcinogenic dose. The second stage called promotion results from repeated application of specific agents, promoting agents, which are not carcinogens by themselves. Promoting agents can be defined as damaging materials capable of causing tumorigenesis only in those cells that have been modified genetically by a carcinogen. The most widely used promoting agent is 12-0-tetradecanoyl-phorbol-13-acetate (TPA), which has been purified from croton oil by Hecker (13) and Van Duuren (14). It was noted that the action of the promoter was successfully blocked by synthetic protease inhibitors, anti-inflammatory hormones and retinoids (15-17). Several distinct stages of promotion were specifically blocked by these agents (18).

In early studies, the pure protease inhibitors TLCK, TPCK (19) and leupeptin (2) were applied topically to block tumor formation on skin. More recently, rats fed a soybean diet were protected against X-ray induced breast tumors (21). This work has stimulated a new look at protease and protease inhibitors in relation to carcinogenesis. Several laboratories have shown that protease inhibitors block in vitro transformation in 10T½ cells and that soybean trypsin inhibitor (Kunitz) blocks the promotional effect of TPA on in vitro transformation (22,23).

Tumor promoters are responsible for the wide variety of reactions in cells, but the exact mechanism by which the tumor promoter acts in inducing tumors is still unknown. One possible mechanism with which we favor is that the damage caused by tumor promoters is in part due to the formation of free oxygen radicals, resulting from perturbation of the cell membrane of polymorpho nucleosides (PMNs) and macrophages. Inhibitors of tumor promotion described for the mouse skin model, such as protease inhibitors, steroids and retinoids, also counteract superoxide anion formation in PMNs (24,25,26).

Recently, Slaga reported that in addition to the phorbol ester tumor promoters, benzoyl peroxide, a widely used free radical-generating compound, is an effective tumor promoter in mouse skin. Moreover, he found that the antioxidants butylated hydroxyl anisol (BHA) and butylated hydroxytoluene (BHT) are potent inhibitors of TPA promotion (27).

Soybean diets rich in protease inhibitors in comparison to casein diets devoid of protease inhibitors protect experimental animals from tumor formation. This was observed in two stage skin carcinogenesis in mice (28), in X-ray induced breast cancer in rats (21) and spontaneous liver cancer in mice (29). A synthetic protease inhibitor ε-amino-caproic acid supplied in the drinking water of experimental animals has been shown to block dimethyl hydrazine induced colon cancer in mice (30). In order to learn the mechanism of the effect of ingested proteases we studied the metabolic fate of ingested Bowman-Birk inhibitor of soybeans.

Metabolic Fate of Protease Inhibitors

Soybeans contain two types of proteinase inhibitors: Bowman-Birk and Kunitz. Bowman-Birk (BB) represents a family of inhibitors present in all legumes, whereas the Kunitz inhibitor is peculiar to soybeans (31). The BB inhibitors are extensively disulfide bonded, acid resistant and stable to food processing (32). Studies using diets supplemented with BB or Kunitz inhibitors demonstrated lower intestinal protease activity only in BB-treated animals (33). Moreover, immunoreactive $[^{125}I]BB$ has been detected in the intestinal tract and feces of chicks (34). We have studied the distribution of $[^{125}I]BB$ in rodents and observed biochemically active BB in the intestinal tract. Over 90% of the inhibitor was located in feces and the colon.

Two mechanisms whereby ingested legumes, rich in pro- tease inhibitors, could act as dietary anticarcinogens may involve 1) a direct effect of protease inhibitors particu- larly applicable to colon cancer; and 2) an indirect effect of protease inhibitors on protein digestion and absorption, thus affecting the nutritional status of the animal.

Preparation of ^{125}I Bowman-Birk Inhibitor

BB inhibitor was prepared from soybean powder following the method of Birk (35). Iodination using $Na(^{125}I)$ obtained from New England Nuclear was performed by the lacto peroxi- dase method. $Na(^{125}I)$ was removed on a Sephadex G-25 column. The $(^{125}I)BB$ was purified by chromatography on a chymotrypsin Sepharose column (36) equilibrated with 0.01 M phosphate, pH 7.4. Inhibitor was dissociated by elution pH 2.6. The specific activity of $(^{125}I)BB$ was of the order of 10 μCi/mg protein.

High performance liquid chromatography (HPLC) was per- formed using a Gilson HPLC system equipped with a TSK-2000 column equilibrated and eluted at 1 ml/min with 0.05 M phosphate, 0.1 M NaCl, pH 7.4. One-minute fractions were collected and counted in an LKB gamma counter.

Proteinase $[^{125}I]BB$ Complex Formation and Dissociation

Complex formation was achieved by mixing 1 mg/ml tryp- sin or chymotrypsin (Worthington) in 0.05 M phosphate,

0.1 M NaCl, pH 7.4 with [125I]BB at room temperature (25°C)
for 15 minutes. Complexes were dissociated by incubating
samples at pH 2.6, room temperature (25°C) for 15 minutes.
Precipitates generated during acid were removed by centri-
fuging samples in a Beckman microfuge for 5 minutes. Analysis of products was achieved by HPLC and counting fractions.
Sample volume loaded on HPLC was 400 µl.

This method provides a rapid method of determining
biological activity of [125I]BB, providing the molecular
weight of the radioactive material occurring in biological
material and noting a change when trypsin or chymotrypsin
is added and complexes with active inhibitor. Moreover,
protease/inhibitor complex can be diagnosed by noting dissociation in acid forming the free inhibitor with the
expected mol. wt. 16.000. The protease/inhibitor complex
has the molecular weight of 33.000, with BB inhibitor contributing 8000 the protease about 25.000. The property of
inhibitor to form complexes with proteases demonstrates its
biological activity.

Animal Experiments

Five-week-old male Sprague-Dawley rats were fasted for
18 hours prior to administration of [125I]BB. Animals were
lightly anesthetized with ether and administered the [125I]BB
(0.001 - 0.1 mg, 10^4 - 10^6 cpm in 0.1 ml phosphate buffered
saline) with a gavaging needle (Popper and Sons, New Hyde
Park, NY). Rats were sacrificed after 1, 2, 3, 4 and 5 hours.
Organs were removed and counted. Distribution of radioactivity was determined as a percent of total radioactivity
recovered. Recovery ranged from 65-100% with no difference
in percent distribution. [125I]plasminogen was administered
to rats and tissues processed as for the [125I]BB treated
animals.

Five-week-old male C3H/HEN mice were divided into three
groups. Prior to administration of [125I]BB, one group was
fasted for 18 hours, a second group was fed Purina Chow and
a third group was fed Purina Chow and 2 mg/ml unlabeled BB
was administered with [125I]BB. All animals were given 1 x
10^6 cpm [125I]BB by gavage. After one hour, animals were
sacrificed and organs removed and counted.

Tissues and feces were homogenized in 0.05 M phosphate,
0.01 M NaCl, pH 7.4, and centrifuged in a Beckman microfuge

prior to chromatography on TSK-2000 and/or chymotrypsin-sepharose.

Distribution of [^{125}I]BB and [^{125}I]Plasminogen in Rats and Mice

Eighteen-hour-fasted rats were administered labeled proteins by gavage and sacrificed after various times. Tissues were dissected and counted. [^{125}I]BB rapidly passes through the stomach and radioactivity accumulates in the colon and feces (74-92% distribution after 1 and 5 hours, respectively). Total recovery ranged from 65-100% and in all cases the percent distribution of [^{125}I]BB from each animal was similar. As an internal control, the lungs of all animals were counted to control for errors in gavage. The counts accumulated in urine (6.2 - 3.5% after 2 and 5 hours, respectively) was to less than 1% of that in other tissues.

Distribution of [^{125}I]plasminogen, as an example of a more typical protein, was also assessed and revealed a significantly different distribution pattern from [^{125}I]BB after 5 hours. [^{125}I]plasminogen passed more slowly through the stomach (30% vs. 2% [^{125}I]plasminogen vs. [^{125}I]BB, respectively), and significant radioactivity was detected in the urine (30% vs. 3% labeled plasminogen vs. BB, respectively). The distribution of labeled plasminogen was 30% vs. 92% in the labeled BB treated animals in the feces.

Distribution of labeled BB in mice was similar to rats. BB accumulated in the intestinal tract and feces regardless of whether animals were fed, fasted or administered [^{125}I]BB with 2 mg unlabeled inhibitor.

Characterization of Ingested [^{125}I]BB

High performance liquid chromatography of feces extracts from rats after 2 and 3 hours of exposure to [^{125}I]BB were performed. After 2 hours the feces contained ^{125}I eluting with an apparent molecular weight of 33,000 daltons. This is the precise elution position of [^{125}I]BB complexed with trypsin or chymotrypsin, demonstrating that BB is combined with a protease. Chromatography of the feces extract acidified to pH 2.5 (conditions known to dissociate protease-BB complexes) revealed a broad peak eluting in a position coincident with the [^{125}I]BB starting material –

16,000 daltons.

Mouse feces was characterized using both HPLC and affinity chromatography. HPLC data were similar to rats in that material eluted at an apparent molecular weight consistent with complex formation and was dissociable into a broad peak or radioactivity eluting as labeled BB starting material.

Conclusion

We have determined the metabolic fate of ingested BB inhibitor and assessed its biochemical activity using HPLC and affinity chromatography. The [^{125}I]BB administered orally to mice and rats distributed almost exclusively into the intestinal tract and feces. This is in agreement with distribution of labeled BB in chicks (34). The low recovery of immunoreactive BB in chicks may be due to BB complexing with proteases. The distribution is consistent with the interpretation that BB is not digested and absorbed into the bloodstream. The small percent of ingested BB which is absorbed and concentrated in the urine fails to bind to trypsin or chymotrypsin.

Characterization of labeled BB in feces demonstrated a peak of ^{125}I eluting as a 33,000 dalton material. We have not identified the material to which BB is associated; however, it is most likely BB complexed with protease for the following reasons: 1) The molecular weight is consistent with a complex between a 25,000 dalton serine protease and an 8,000 dalton inhibitor (BB); 2) Complexes between purified trypsin or chymotrypsin and labeled BB prepared in vitro elute as a 33,000 dalton material; 3) Labeled BB starting material can be regenerated from the "complex" when treated under conditions known to dissociate protease/BB inhibitor complexes. Affinity chromatography on chymotrypsin-sepharose columns confirms HPLC data which suggests that BB is capable of binding protease. Thus, BB inhibitor does not become degraded in the stomach and enters the intestine as an unchanged biochemically active protein.

The Bowman-Birk inhibitor is an 8,000 dalton protein, however, it occurs as a 16,000 dalton dimer in solution. Upon complexing with protease, the dimer dissociates and a complex is formed with a molecular weight consistent with a 1:1 protease:protease inhibitor complex.

Protease inhibitors, as presented by the Bowman-Birk soybean trypsin inhibitor, can escape the usual digestive route of proteins and appear fully active in the duodenum where they may inhibit the absorption of other proteins. The precise mechanism remains unclear; however, one possibility is that complexes between protease and inhibitors may remove some of the trypsin and chymotrypsin for the digestion of other proteins, thus contributing to decreased protein absorption. High protein intake has been identified as one of the necessary conditions for carcinogenesis (Campbell, personal communication). Thus, decreased absorption of proteins may be in part responsible for the anticarcinogenic action of protease inhibitors. In the case of colon carcinogenesis, dietary proteinase inhibitors may act directly as an anticarcinogen because of the high concentration of the inhibitor there. The demonstration that a synthetic inhibitor given in the water supply to mice successfully blocks colon carcinogenesis (30) makes this a promising lead to pursue in proposing nutritional alteration in preventing colon cancer to feed legume seeds rich in BB type of protease inhibitor. The anticarcinogenic action of protease inhibitors in the diet of skin, breast and liver cancer in animal experiments (28, 21, 29) and human epidemyological data in breast and prostatic cancer (9) may present inhibition of protein digestion as the underlying mechanism. Further work in the precise distribution and action of protease inhibitors in vivo is required to confirm this mechanism. The combined action of protease inhibitors and other blockers of tumor promotion in particular retinoids present important opportunities for intervention of nutrition in prevention of cancer.

Bibliography

1. Ryan, C.A. (1973). Ann. Rev. Plant Physiol. 24:173.
2. Carp, H., Janoff, A. (1978). Ann Rev. Respir. Dis. 118: 617.
3. Janoff, A., White, R., Carp, H., Harel, S., Dearing, R., Lee, D.K. (1979). Ann. J. Pathol. 97:111.
4. Janoff, A., Carp, H., Lee, D.K., Drew, R.T. (1979). Science 206.
5. Clark, R.A., Stone, P.J., Hag, A.E., Calore, J.D., Franzblau, C. (1981). J. Biol. Chem. 256:3348.
6. Meyn, M.S., Rossman, R., Troll, W. (1977). Proc. Natl. Acad. Sci. USA 74:1152-1156.

7. Phillips, R.L. (1975). Cancer Res. 35:3513.
8. Armstrong, B., Doll, R. (1975). Int. J. Cancer 15:617.
9. Correa, P. (1981). Cancer Res. 41:3685
10. Carroll, K.K. (1975). Cancer Res. 35:3374.
11. Berenblum, I., Shubik, P. (1947). Br. J. Cancer 1:383.
12. Boutwell, R.K. (1964). Prog. Exp. Tumor Res. 4:207.
13. Hecker, E. (1966). Proc. IX Int. Cancer Congr., Tokyo, Abstract p. 17.
14. Van Duuren, B.L. (1969). Prog. Exp. Tumor Res. 11:31.
15. Troll, W. (1976). In: Fundamentals in Cancer Prevention, P.N. Magee, S. Takayama, T. Sugimura, and T. Matsushima, eds., p. 41.
16. Belman, S., Troll, W. (1972). Cancer Res. 32:450.
17. Verma, A.K., Boutwell, R.K. (1977). Cancer Res. 37: 196.
18. Slaga, T.J., Klein-Szanto, J.P., Fischer, S.M., Weeks, C.E., Nelson, K., Major, S. (1980). Proc. Natl. Acad. Sci. 77:2251.
19. Troll, W., Klassen, A., Janoff, A. (1971). Science 169: 1211.
20. Hozumi, M., Ogawa, M., Sugimura, T., Takeuchi, T., Umezawa, H. (1972). Cancer Res. 32:1725.
21. Troll, W., Wiesner, R., Shellabarger, C.J., Holtzman, S., Stone, J.P. (1980). Carcinogenesis 1:469.
22. Borek, C., Miller, R., Pain, C., Troll, W. (1979). Proc. Natl. Acad. Sci. 76:1800.
23. Kennedy, A.R., Little, J.B. (1981). Cancer Res. 41: 2103.
24. Goldstein, B.D., Witz, G., Amoruso, M., Stone, D.S., Troll, W. (1981). Cancer Lett. 11:257.
25. Witz, G., Goldstein, B.D., Amoruso, M., Stone, D.S., Troll, W. (1980). Biochem. Biophys. Res. Commun. 97: 883.
26. Goldstein, B.D., Witz, G., Amoruso, M., Troll, W. (1979). Biochem. Biophys. Res. Commun. 88:854.
27. Slaga, T.J., Klein-Szanto, A.J.P., Triplett, L.L., Yotti, L.P., Trosko, J.E. (1981). Science (Wash.) 213:1023.
28. Troll, W., Belman, S., Wiesner, R., Shellabarger, C.J. (1979). Protease action in carcinogenesis. In: Biological Function of Proteinases, H. Holzer and H. Tschesche, eds., pp. 165-170.
29. Becker, F.F. (1981). Carcinogenesis 2:1213-1214.
30. Corasanti, J.G., Hobilua, G.H., Marcus, G. (1982). Science 216:1020-1021.

31. Laskowski, M., Jr., Kato, I. (1980). Annu. Rev. Biochem. 49:593-626.
32. Yavelow, J., Gitlund, M., Troll, W. (1982). Carcinogenesis 3:135-138.
33. Gertler, A., Birk, Y., Bondi, A. (1967). J. Nutr. 91:358-370.
34. Madar, Z., Gertler, A., Birk, Y. (1979). Comp. Biochem. Physiol. 62A:1057-1061.
35. Birk, Y. (1961). Biochim. Biophys. Acta. 54:378-381.
36. Finlay, T.H., Troll, V., Levy, M., Johnson, A.J., Hodgkin, L.T. (1978). Analy. Biochem. 87:77-90.

Acknowledgment

This work was supported by a grant from the U.S. Public Health Service, grant number CA 16060.

Diet, Nutrition, and Cancer:
From Basic Research to Policy Implications, pages 177–194
© *1983 Alan R. Liss, Inc., 150 Fifth Avenue, New York, NY 10011*

MUTAGENS IN COOKED BEEF: CHARACTERIZATION AND GENOTOXIC
EFFECTS

James S. Felton, Frederick T. Hatch, Mark G.
Knize, and Leonard F. Bjeldanes*
Biomedical Sciences Division, Lawrence
Livermore National Laboratory, University of
California, Livermore, CA 94550 and *Department
of Nutritional Sciences, Berkeley, CA

ABSTRACT

Recently a number of laboratories, including our own,
have been concerned with identifying and characterizing
genotoxic substances produced during the cooking of foods
(especially beef), and the relationship of these substances
to the incidence of cancer of the gastrointestinal tract.
We have developed an efficient extraction procedure incorporating XAD resin adsorption, which when applied to grilled
ground beef, yields an extract showing 230 Salmonella
TA 1538 revertants per gram fresh weight of original ground
beef. The mutagenic components of the beef are specific
for frameshift-sensitive Salmonella strains, and have an
absolute requirement for metabolic activation. This
activation with rat or mouse liver systems was greatest
with cytochrome P-448 type of metabolism. Human liver
microsomes and flavonoid-induced rodent intestinal S9 were
also active metabolizing fractions. The mutagenic material
from ground beef, when further fractionated by low- and
high-pressure liquid chromatography, resulted in two major
and a few minor active fractions. One of the major fractions has been identified as (2-amino-3,8-dimethylimidazo-
[4,5f]quinoxaline (MeIQ$_x$).

Analysis of the major sources of cooked protein intake
in the American diet (based on U.S.D.A. and U.S.D.H.E.W.
surveys) showed significant mutagen content in beef, eggs,
pork, ham, and bacon, and a somewhat lower amount in chicken
and fish after being fried or broiled well-done. Tofu,

beans, cheese, and some fish, when heated under similar cooking conditions, produced low or negligible mutagenic activity.

Two potent bacterial mutagens thermally produced in foods, 3-amino-1-methyl-5H-pyrido[4,3-b]indole (Trp-P-2) and 2-amino-3-methylimidazo[4,5-f]quinoline (IQ), were examined in cultured mammalian cells. In excision-repair-deficient Chinese hamster ovary (CHO) cells, Trp-P-2 caused cytotoxicity, mutagenicity (thioguanine and azaadenine resistance), sister chromatid exchange, and chromosomal aberrations at concentrations more than 30-fold lower than those for IQ. In normal repair- proficient CHO cells, Trp-P-2 was one-half as active and IQ was inactive. In contrast, Trp-P-2 is much less potent than IQ in the Salmonella mutagenesis assay. Work is in progress to understand the significance of the weak response of IQ in mammalian cells.

INTRODUCTION

The high incidence of gastrointestinal cancer in many countries has been associated with the eating of cooked protein-containing foods (Sugimura et al., 1977; Gray and Morton, 1981; Grice et al., 1981). The cooking of foods produces at least three classes of genotoxic substances. (1) Polycyclic aromatic hydrocarbons are deposited on the meat following the dripping of fat onto an open flame and the subsequent contact of the generated smoke with the meat (Lijinsky and Shubik, 1964; Rhee and Bratzler, 1970; Panalaks, 1976). (2) When amino acid-containing foods or amino acids themselves are heated at high temperatures (400 to 600°C), extremely mutagenic pyrolysis products are produced (Nagao et al., 1977; Kosuge et al., 1978; Matsumoto et al., 1978; Yoshida et al., 1978). (3) Low-temperature (~ 200°C) cooking or frying has been shown by our laboratory and by others to produce mutagenic components after fairly short periods of heating (Felton et al., 1980a; Felton et al., 1981a; Commoner et al., 1978; Pariza et al., 1979; Spingarn and Weisburger 1979).

Identification of the mutagens in cooked foods has started only recently. Two compounds 2-amino-3-methyl-imidazo[4,5-f]quinoline (IQ) (Spingarn et al., 1980), and

2-amino-3,8-dimethylimidazo[4,5-f]quinoxaline (MeIQ$_x$) (Kasai et al., 1981a,b), have been reported in cooked ground beef. The level of contribution of either IQ or MeIQ$_x$ is not clear. Additional major mutagens are definitely present (this manuscript; Hargraves and Pariza, 1982). We have focused our attention on protein-rich foods cooked to a well-done state, especially meats.

Bacterial test systems: Ames/Salmonella, arabinose resistance, and 8-azaguanine resistance all show very sensitive responses to both IQ and the tryptophan pyrolysis product Trp-P-2. Chinese hamster ovary (CHO) cells respond to Trp-P-2 with substantial cytotoxicity, mutagenesis as measured by both thioguanine (TG) and azaadenine (AA) resistance, and cytogenetic damage. In contrast, these endpoints showed only limited responses to IQ, one of the proposed mutagens in cooked beef.

The genotoxic agents found to date in fried and broiled beef reside in the organic base fraction. Metabolic activation of these materials is required for genotoxic effects, and this activation is mediated by cytochrome P-448 enzymes. Slightly differing findings on metabolism of beef mutagens by human subcellular fractions have been reported by Felton et al., (1980b); Felton and Healy (1982); and Dolara et al., (1980).

Further experiments in mammalian cells will, hopefully, help us better assess the risk to humans. This will be done by examining the kinetics of metabolite formation and disappearance, the covalent binding of mutagens to DNA, and a relevant model intestinal toxicity system. This article is a partial summary of our work on establishing a data base for assessing the risk from ingesting mutagens in cooked foods.

CHARACTERIZATION

Cooking Conditions

Cooking is required to produce mutagens in the basic fraction of hamburger (BFH). Mutagenic components can be extracted from the outer portion of the patty following at least 2 minutes of cooking on each side at cooking surface temperatures of 150°C or higher. All the cooking surfaces tested were capable of causing mutagen formation, although a ceramic surface produced a slower response (Bjeldanes et al., 1982a).

Extracting Mutagenic Activity from Foods

The recovery of mutagenic activity has been described in detail (Bjeldanes et al., 1982b). The earliest described method of isolation of the mutagenic materials, using $(NH_4)_2SO_4$ precipitation (Commoner et al., 1978), has proved very inefficient (almost 10 times less so) compared to extraction with aqueous acid followed by adsorption-elution on XAD-2 resin (see Table 1).

Tester Strain Specificity

The basic fraction of cooked beef has marked specificity towards Ames/Salmonella TA 1537, TA 1538, and TA 98, all frameshift-sensitive tester strains. In contrast (Felton et al., 1981a), the base substitution strains TA 1535 and TA 100 show no significant positive mutagenic response. This degree of almost absolute strain specificity is seldom seen with pure chemicals (J. McCann, personal communication; McCann et al., 1975) and suggests a very specific type of nucleic acid interaction of the components present in the BFH. The acid and neutral fractions of cooked beef were also examined for mutagenicity with all five tester strains. No activity was seen in the acid fraction at exposures to over 180 gram equivalents (gE) (a gram equivalent is the amount of extract equivalent to 1 gram fresh weight of original ground beef), and in the neutral fraction up to 27 gE. In contrast, mutagenicity of the basic fraction is readily detected at an exposure level of 0.5 gE.

Specificity of Metabolic Activation

BFH is mutagenic in the Ames/Salmonella test only when activated by S9 or microsomal monooxygenase(s); the parent compounds are inactive without specific metabolism (Felton et al., 1980b). Mouse, hamster, and rat Aroclor-induced hepatic S9 fractions all metabolize the BFH, with the hamster preparation showing the most activity per mg of protein.

TABLE 1

TA 1538 <u>SALMONELLA</u> ASSAY OF EXTRACTS FROM FOUR
DIFFERENT FRACTIONATION METHODS[1]

Method	No. Revertants per gE[2]
Dilute acid-$(NH_4)_2SO_4$[3]	10-31[4]
Acetone[5]	59
Mixed solvent[6]	98
XAD-2 resin[7]	235

[1] For the three methods in which bases were separated
(Dilute acid $(NH_4)_2SO_4$, acetone, and mixed solvent),
only the basic fractions are shown, since the acid and
neutral fractions had no mutagenic activity.

[2] Number of revertants per gram fresh weight of uncooked
meat (gE) is calculated from the slopes of regression
lines in the linear region of the background-corrected
dose-response data.

[3] Method of Commoner <u>et al</u>. (1978).

[4] Range of two experiments.

[5] Method of Felton <u>et al</u>. (1981a).

[6] $CH_3OH:CH_2Cl_2:H_2O$ (45:45:10, v/v/v).

[7] Rohm/Haas (Philadelphia).

Most important have been the studies using human
microsomes to metabolize the BFH. These microsomes
activate the basic fraction significantly more than
microsomes from uninduced mouse or rat liver. The

microsomes from one individual were nearly as active as
those of the Aroclor-induced mice and rats. The human
metabolism is mediated almost exclusively by cytochrome
P-448 because addition of α-naphthoflavone, an inhibitor
of cytochrome P-448 metabolism, to the reaction mixture
inhibits almost completely the formation of mutagenic
products (Felton and Healy, 1982). This result not only
shows the potential for human liver to activate the
hamburger mutagens, but also suggests that the human
liver mixed function oxygenases (cytochrome P-450s) are
being naturally induced through diet and/or environmental
exposures. Thus, at least one human tissue is capable of
activating the mutagens of cooked beef, a positive factor
for risk assessment.

Genetic Toxicology

     Initial studies of the genotoxicity of partially
purified fractions of cooked hamburger gave equivocal
results (Felton et al., 1980c). This led us to use
purified compounds similar in structure to the organic
amines expected to be found in cooked foods. Two
purified model compounds, Trp-P-2 and IQ, were used.
Both compounds are extremely active in Ames/Salmonella
strain TA 1538 in the presence of rodent liver S9. IQ
was over four-fold more active than Trp-P-2 in producing
mutation and cell killing (Thompson et al., 1982). The
dose range of mutational effects was far below the range
for toxicity. In addition, the dependence on lack of a
uvr repair pathway was clear; Salmonella strain TA 1978
(uvrB$^+$) was approximately 100-fold less sensitive.
This difference between the standard and the
repair-sufficient strains indicates that the lesions
produced by Trp-P-2 and IQ are potentially repairable.

     Both compounds were also assessed in our laboratory
for their mutagenicity in two bacterial forward mutation
assays in order to determine if the extremely high
sensitivity and specificity of the Ames histidine-
reversion assay is unique or generally applicable. In
both the arabinose-resistance assay (Whong et al., 1981)
and the 8-azaguanine-resistance assay (Skopek et al.,
1978), Trp-P-2 and IQ were positive, with induced
mutation frequencies similar to those seen in TA 1538.
As in the standard Salmonella assay, IQ was several-fold

more potent than Trp-P-2. A major surprise was the different behavior of the two compounds in the CHO mammalian mutagenesis system. Trp-P-2 was very active at doses more than 100-fold lower than IQ. IQ, even at the highest doses used (limit of solubility), killed only 50% of the cells; and mutation levels were only barely significant. Parallel cytogenetic experiments measuring SCE, chromosomal aberrations and micronuclei, and utilizing the same exposed cell cultures, resulted in sensitivity and dose response curves similar to the mammalian cell mutagenesis experiments (Thompson et al., 1982).

The different (reversed) responses of Trp-P-2 and IQ in CHO cells could be due to either more efficient repair of the DNA lesions induced by IQ, although the UV-5 cells (a strain deficient in UV repair) showed a weak mutagenic response, or to lack of uptake of the activated form of IQ into the cell nucleus. The latter might be due to inactivation of the mutagen in the cytoplasm of the cells by either detoxification pathways or reaction with cellular macromolecules. Binding studies with tritium-labeled IQ (a gift of A. Waterhouse and H. Rapoport, University of California, Berkeley) have begun to determine how much mutagen actually binds to the DNA in these cells. Preliminary experiments (L. Thompson, personal communication) at approximately 50% survival show a fairly high mutagenic efficiency (induced mutations per adduct): 3.2×10^{-9} compared to 7-bromomethylbenz-(a)anthracene (BMBA) (8.1×10^{-10}), a strong mutagen in CHO cells and an animal carcinogen. The absolute amounts of IQ binding to DNA are much less than for BMBA, but the result indicates that if IQ binds, mutations can result. Further experiments are in progress to understand the reactivity of the metabolic intermediates of IQ.

Chemical Isolation and Identification

The most efficient extraction method, aqueous acid solubilization and XAD-2 resin trapping (see above), was used for purifying the mutagenic components (organic amines) (Kasai et al., 1981b) from a 3.5-kg batch of fried ground beef patties. A preparative reverse-phase high-pressure liquid chromatography (HPLC) separation (20% acetonitrile-H_2O) gave two distinct mutagenic

activities: RpI and RpII. They contained 59 and 41% of
the mutagenic activity, respectively (Data not shown).
The RpI activity, when rechromatographed on HPLC with
normal phase separation (17.5% n-propanol in hexane
through two Nagel NH_2 columns), gave two well-separated
peaks with mutagenic activity: early normal phase and
late normal phase (Fig. 1a). Neither peak co-eluted with
IQ or MeIQ standards. Each peak was then rerun on a
reverse phase column, resulting in clearly different
fractions with coincident UV absorbance and Salmonella
activity. The early-normal phase peak (the less polar of
the two) does not co-elute with any known standards
(Fig. 1b), and is being analyzed with mass spectroscopy.
The more polar late-normal phase peak (Fig. 1c) has the
ultraviolet spectral properties and specific activity
(revertants/A unit) of $MeIQ_x$ (Kasai et al., 1981b). By
mass spectrometry the molecular ion m/e 213 is identical
to $MeIQ_x$, with fragment ions at m/e 212, m/e 197,
m/e 185, and m/e 144. This component is approximately 40
to 50% of the total recovered mutagenic activity (for
Salmonella) in the hamburger. The RpII activity was more
difficult to purify, as it co-eluted on a normal phase
column with a large UV peak (Fig. 2a). This component
when rechromatographed under reverse phase conditions
(Fig. 2b) appears to be 30-40% of the total mutagenic
activity of the hamburger. Further purification and
identification are underway. No known standards co-elute
with this mutagenic activity.

A larger batch (40 kg) of ground beef is being
processed at this time. The amounts of purified material
should be sufficient for NMR and high-resolution mass
spectroscopy, so that structural identification can be
made on the two unidentified mutagenic components (RpI
early normal phase fraction, and RpII).

Food Survey

The formation of mutagens in the major cooked
protein-rich foods in the U.S. diet was studied. The
nine cooked protein-containing foods most commonly eaten
(ground beef, beefsteak, eggs, pork chops, fried chicken,
pot roast, ham, roast beef, and bacon were determined by
Plumlee et al., (1981) from the U.S.D.A. and U.S.D.H.E.W.
surveys and were examined for their mutagenic activity in

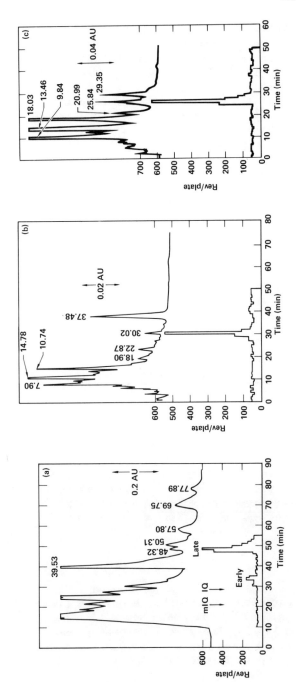

Figure 1. HPLC separation of two preparative reverse phase activity fractions (early and late RpI peaks). a) Normal phase separation using two 30 cm amine columns (Macherey-Nagel, Germany) in series. Separation was isocratic with 17.5% n-propanol and 0.1% acetic acid in hexane. Flow was 1.0 ml/min. b) Analytical reverse phase separation of early normal phase activity peak with a 25 cm partisil 5 μm ODS-3 column (Whatman, Clifton, NJ). Separation was isocratic with 30% MeOH and 0.1% diethylamine in H2O. c) Analytical reverse phase separation of late normal phase activity peak (conditions same as b). In a, b, and c rev/plate are the result of plating 1% of each 1 min fraction with TA 1538 and S9 from Aroclor treated rats.

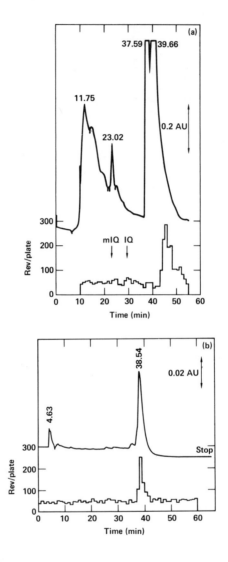

Figure 2. HPLC separation of preparative reverse phase
II activity fraction. a) Normal phase separation as
described in Figure 1. b) Analytical reverse phase
separation as described in Figure 1. Rev/plate are
calculated as described in Figure 1.

TA 1538 following extraction by the acetone method (see Table 2). Multiplying the number of revertants per gE by the average daily portion consumed in grams will give the average daily revertant intake in the diet if foods are cooked well done. The total of the right-hand column is about 5600 revertants. We have also found mutagen equal to as many as 5,900 revertants in a commercially cooked hamburger (Bjeldanes et al., 1982c). Since the acetone method extracts only 25% of the mutagens from the ground beef (Bjeldanes et al., 1982b), we have made the assumption in Table 2 that the efficiency would be similar in the other eight foods (pending direct measurement with the XAD method). Thus the total revertant intake should be at least 22,500 Ames/Salmonella revertants per day in the average American diet if cooked well done. This is equivalent to the ingested mutagenic activity of at least five cigarettes (Sugimura, 1979). Approximately 25% (4000 Salmonella revertants) of the total mutagenic material in a cigarette is retained in the lung. In another comparison, cooked foods have 200 times the mutagenic activity of aflatoxin B_1 in the American diet from corn and peanuts (Hsieh, 1982). The latter value is calculated from a 5.6 ng/man/day exposure and an aflatoxin B_1 mutagenicity of 22 revertants/ng (McCann et al., 1975) resulting in an intake of 123 revertants/man/day.

In addition, other types of protein-containing foods (not necessarily the main sources of protein in the U.S.) were examined (see Table 3). The principal meats, beef, pork, etc., showed the highest mutagen content. Chicken and fish were intermediate, and beans, tofu, and cheese were very low or at background levels.

The different modes of cooking gave large variations in mutagen formation (Bjeldanes, 1982c,d). Broiling, grilling (frying), and high-temperature baking produced large numbers of revertants, while stewing, braising, deep frying, or low-temperature baking gave very small numbers or none above background. It seems clear that all major protein-rich foods, if cooked well-done (200°C or hotter), except eggs (which must be cooked at over 225°C), will contain bacterial mutagens.

Table 2

INGESTION OF MUTAGEN IN THE AVERAGE AMERICAN DIET
FOLLOWING NORMAL (WELL-DONE) COOKING METHODS

Major Protein Foods	Mutagenicity in TA1538 (Revertants/ gE)	Average Daily Food Intake Fresh Weight (g/d)	Mutagen Ingested (Revertants/Day)
Ground beef[1]	63.0	30.5	1920
Beef steak[1]	40.0	32.2	1290
Eggs[2]	12.4	31.0	390
Pork chops[1]	42.0	9.8	410
Fried chicken[3]	11.8	17.2	200
Beef, braised or pot roast[4]	0.70	6.6	5
Ham[1]	51.0	13.0	660
Roast beef[5]	35.5	13.8	470
Bacon[1]	20.5	13.2	270
			Total 5615 Rev/day

[1] Fried 6 min/side at initial pan temperature of 200°C.

[2] Fried 4 min/side at 275°C.

[3] Deep fried 23 min at 101°C.

[4] Oven-heated 135 min at 100°C.

[5] Oven-roasted 90 min at 176°C.

Table 3

COMPARATIVE MUTAGENICITIES OF DIFFERENT PROTEIN SOURCES FOLLOWING FRYING

	Temperature	Time (min per side)	No. Revertants per 100 gE[1]
Beef (hamburger)	200	6	6300
Pork (ham)	200	6	6000
Chicken (white meat)	103	12.5	1000
Fish (rock cod)	200	6	1334
Eggs	225	6	171
Beans (kidney)[2]	200	8	147
Tofu	150	6	69
Cheese (american)	300	5	63

[1] Revertants of strain TA1538 calculated as in Table 1 (mean spontaneous revertant rate for all eight experiments is 24).

[2] Beans were boiled first for 45 minutes and were fried for a total of 8 min.

CONCLUSIONS

Optimum conditions for extraction of mutagens from ground beef have been achieved. A number of mutagenic fractions are seen with one of the major being identified as $MeIQ_x$. The mutagens present in the ground beef are specific for causing frameshift mutations and are metabolized to active intermediates by cytochrome P-448. This specific activation is also seen in human liver as well as rodent liver and intestine.

The major sources of protein in the American diet when cooked well-done and maximally extracted from the food can result in ingested mutagenic components with Salmonella activity over 20,000 revertants per day. This mutagenic exposure is equivalent to the retained genotoxic activity of approximately 5 cigarettes. Compared to aflatoxin B_1, the well-done foods contribute 200 times more mutagenic (Salmonella) material to the daily human exposure in the U.S.

The significance of the weak response of IQ, one of two standard food related mutagens used in the comparative gentoxicity studies, in mammalian systems is not well understood at this time. Binding studies indicate very little reactive IQ binds the DNA of CHO cells following exogenous S9 activation. But what does reach the nucleus appears potent at producing genetic changes. More work (i.e., whole animal carcinogenicity and additional mammalian cell analysis) clearly needs to be done to develop a good data base from which reasonable human risk extrapolations can be made.

ACKNOWLEDGMENTS

Work performed under the auspices of the U.S. Department of Energy by the Lawrence Livermore National Laboratory under contract number W-7405-ENG-48 and supported by an Interagency Agreement (NIEHS 222Y01-ES-10063) between the National Institute of Environmental Health Sciences and the Department of Energy. The authors would like to thank S. Healy, M. Morris, C. Morris, and T. Wood for their fine technical contributions.

REFERENCES

Ames BN, McCann J, Yamasaki E (1975). Methods for detecting carcinogens and mutagens with the Salmonella/ mammalian-microsome mutagenicity test. Mutation Res 31:347-364.

Bjeldanes LF, Morris M, Timourian H, Hatch FT (1982a).
Effects of meat composition and cooking conditions on
mutagen formation in fried ground beef. J Agric and Food
Chem (in press).

Bjeldanes LF, Grose KR, Davis PH, Stuermer DH, Healy SK,
Felton JS (1982b). An XAD-2 resin method for efficient
extraction of mutagens from fried ground beef. Mutation
Res Lett (in press).

Bjeldanes LF, Morris MM, Felton JS, Healy S, Stuermer D,
Berry P, Timourian H, Hatch FT (1982c). Mutagens from
the cooking of food II. Survey of mutagen formation in
the major protein-rich foods of the North American diet.
Food Chem Toxicol (in press).

Bjeldanes LF, Morris MM, Felton JS, Healy S, Stuermer D,
Berry P, Timourian H, Hatch FT (1982d). Mutagens from
the cooking of food III. Secondary sources of cooked
dietary protein. Food Chem Toxicol (in press).

Commoner B, Vithayathil AJ, Dolara P, Nair S, Madyastha
P, Cuca GC (1978). Formation of mutagens in beef and
beef extract during cooking. Science 201:913-916.

Dolara P, Barale R, Mazzoli S, Benetti D (1980).
Activation of the mutagens of beef extract *in vitro* and
in vivo. Mutat Res 79:213-221.

Felton J, Healy S, Stuermer D, Berry C, Timourian H,
Hatch F, Bjeldanes L, Morris M (1980a). Improved
isolation and characterization of mutagenic fractions
from cooked ground beef. Environ Mutag 2:304.

Felton JS, Healy SK, Orwig DS, Stuermer DH, Berry PW,
Timourian H, Hatch FT, Bjeldanes LF, Morris M (1980b).
Metabolism of mutagenic fractions from cooked ground
beef. Proc Amer Assoc Cancer Res 21:125.

Felton J, Carrano AV, Carver J, Thompson L, Stuermer D,
Timourian H, Hatch F, Bjeldanes L, Morris M (1980c).
Evaluation of mutagens from cooked hamburger with several
short-term mammalian bioassays. Environ Mutag 2:303-304.

Felton JS, Healy S, Stuermer D, Berry C, Timourian H, Hatch FT, Morris M, Bjeldanes LF (1981a). Mutagens from the cooking of food I. Improved isolation and characterization of mutagenic fractions from cooked ground beef. Mutation Res 88:33-44.

Felton JS, Healy SK, Knize M, Stuermer DH, Berry PW, Timourian H, Hatch FT, Morris M, Bjeldanes LF (1981b). In vitro human and rodent metabolism of mutagenic fractions from cooked ground beef. Environ Mutag 3:342.

Felton JS, Healy SK (1982). Mutagenic activation of cooked ground beef by human liver microsomes. Science (submitted).

Gray JI, Morton ID (1981). Some toxic compounds produced in food by cooking and processing. J Hum Nutr, 35:5-23.

Grice HC, Clegg DJ, Coffin DE, Lo M-T, Middleton EJ, Sandi E, Scott PM, Sen NP, Smith BL, Withey JR (1981). Carcinogens in foods. In Sontag JM (ed): "Carcinogens in Industry and the Environment," New York and Basel, Marcel Dekker, Inc., Chapt. 10.

Hargraves WA, Pariza MW (1982). Purification and characterization of bacterial mutagens from commercial beef extract and fried ground beef. Proc Amer Assoc Cancer Res 23: 92.

Hatch FT, Felton JS, Bjeldanes LF (1982). Mutagens from the cooking of food: Thermic mutagens in beef. In Stich H, Powrie W (eds): "Carcinogens and Mutagens in Food, Critical Reviews of Toxicology," Boca Raton, CRC Press (in press).

Hayatsu H, Inoue K, Ohta H, Namba T, Togawa K, Hayatsu T, Makita M, Wataya Y (1981). Inhibition of the mutagenicity of cooked beef basic fraction by its acidic fraction. Mutation Res 91:437-442.

Hsieh D (1982). These proceedings.

Kasai H, Shiomi T, Sugimura T, Nishimura S (1981a). Synthesis of 2-amino-3,8-dimethylimidazo[4,5-f] quinoxaline (Me-IQx), a potent mutagen isolated from fried beef. Chemistry Lett 675-678.

Kąsai H, Yamaizumi Z, Shiomi T, Yokoyama S, Miyazawa T, Wakabayashi K, Nagao M, Sugimura T, Nishimura S (1981b). Structure of a potent mutagen isolated from fried beef. Chemistry Lett 485-488.

Kosuge T, Tsuji K, Wakabayashi K, Okamoto T, Shudo K, Iitaka Y, Itai A, Sugimura T, Kawachi T, Nagao M, Yahagi T, Seino Y (1978). Isolation and structure studies of mutagenic principles in amino acid pyrolysates. Chem Pharm Bull 26(2):611.

Lijinsky W, Shubik P (1964). Benzo(a)pyrene and other polynuclear hydrocarbons in charcoal-broiled meat. Science 145:53-55.

McCann J, Choi E, Yamasaki E, Ames BN (1975). Detection of carcinogens in Salmonella/microsome tests: Assay of 300 chemicals. Proc Natl Acad Sci USA 72:5135-5139.

Matsumoto T, Yoshida D, Mizusaki S, Okamoto H (1978). Mutagenicities of the pyrolysates of peptides and proteins. Mutation Res 56:281-288.

Nagao M, Honda M, Seino Y, Yahagi T, Sugimura T (1977). Mutagenicities of smoke condensates and the charred surface of fish and meat. Cancer Lett 2:221-226.

Panalaks T (1976). Determination and identification of polycyclic aromatic hydrocarbons in smoked and charcoal-broiled food products by high pressure liquid chromatography and gas chromatography. J Environ Sci Health B11:299-315.

Pariza MW, Ashoor SH, Chu FS, Lund DB (1979). Effects of temperature and time on mutagen formation in pan-fried hamburger. Cancer Lett 7:63-69.

Pezzuto J, Moore P, Hecht S (1981). Metabolic activation of 1-methyl-3-amino-5H-pyrido[4,3-b] indole and several structurally related mutagens. Biochemistry 20:298-305.

Plumlee C, Bjeldanes LF, Hatch FT (1981). Food item priority assessment for studies of mutagen production during cooking. J Am Dietet Assoc 79:201-204.

Rhee KS, Bratzler LJ (1970). Benzo(a)pyrene in smoked meat products. J Food Sci 35:146-149.

Skopek TR, Leber HL, Krolewski JJ, Thilly WC (1978). Quantitative forward mutation assay in Salmonella typhimurium using 8-azaguanine resistance as a genetic marker. Proc Natl Acad Sci USA 75:410-414.

Spingarn NE, Weisburger JH (1979). Formation of mutagens in cooked food. I: Beef. Cancer Lett 7:259-264.

Spingarn NE, Kasai H, Vuolo LL, Nishimura S, Yamaizumi Z, Sugimura T, Matsushima T, Weisburger JH (1980). Formation of mutagens in cooked foods. III: Isolation of a potent mutagen from beef. Cancer Lett 9:177-183.

Sugimura T, Nagao M, Kawachi T, Honda M, Yahagi T, Seino Y, Sato S, Matsukura N, Matsushima T, Shirai A, Sawamura M, Matsumoto H (1977). Mutagen-carcinogens in foods with special reference to highly mutagenic pyrolytic products in broiled foods. In Hiatt HH, Watson JD, Winsten JA (eds): "Origins of Human Cancer," Cold Spring Harbor Lab, pp 1561-1577.

Sugimura T (1979). Naturally occurring genotoxic carcinogens. In: Miller EC et al., (eds): "Naturally Occurring Carcinogen-Mutagens and Modulators of Carcinogenesis," Tokyo and Baltimore, Japan Sci Soc Press and Univ Park Press, pp 241-261.

Thompson LH, Carrano AV, Salazar E, Felton JS, Hatch FT (1982). Comparative genotoxic effects of the cooked-food-related mutagens Trp-P-2 and IQ in bacteria and cultured mammalian cells. Mutation Res (in press).

Whong WZ, Stewart J, Ong TM (1981). Use of the improved arabinose-resistant assay system of Salmonella typhimurium for mutagenesis testing. Environ Mutagen 3:95-99.

Yoshida D, Matsumoto T, Yoshimura R, Matsuzaki T (1978). Mutagenicity of amino-α-carbolines in pyrolysis products of soybean globulin. Biochemical and Biophysical Res Comm 83(3):915-920.

RISK ASSESSMENT: EXPERIMENTAL AND EPIDEMIOLOGICAL

Diet, Nutrition, and Cancer:
From Basic Research to Policy Implications, pages 197–201
© *1983 Alan R. Liss, Inc., 150 Fifth Avenue, New York, NY 10011*

OVERVIEW

DAVID SCHOTTENFELD, M.D.

Chief of Epidemiology & Preventive Medicine
Memorial Sloan-Kettering Cancer Center
New York, NY   10021

Much human cancer is now believed to result from exposure to environmental chemicals, and although the mechanisms
of carcinogenesis are still not fully understood, various
experimental models and observational epidemiologic studies have supported the view of a multistage process. The
notion that nutritional factors may serve either to enhance
or inhibit the level of risk or tumor incidence and time of
appearance of tumors or latency is not a new concept, but
one that is emerging with greater clarity.

International comparisons of site-specific mortality,
and the "experiments of nature" provided by migrant studies,
have suggested that certain features of the Western diet
contribute to a significant but uncertain proportion of all
cancers, and in particular cancers of the large intestine,
pancreas, breast, ovary, endometrium, and prostate. Various
estimates have been made of the proportion of human cancer
incidence that may be attributed to diet. Wynder and Gori
(1977) concluded that a little more than 40% of cancers in
men and almost 60% of cancers in women in the United States
could be attributed to dietary factors.

Doll and Peto (1981) agreed that a substantial proportion of cancers in both sexes in the United States was attributable to dietary factors. They estimated that through
dietary modifications, we might ultimately achieve a 35%
reduction in cancer mortality in the United States. Potentially, they inferred that this overall reduction would em-
brace 90% of large bowel and stomach cancer mortality, 50%
of breast and endometrial cancer mortality, and 20% of lung,

oral cavity, and urinary bladder cancer mortality. These extrapolations were derived from epidemiologic studies which yielded estimations of relative risk and population attributable risk, and from viewing the extremes of site-specific cancer incidence and mortality rates throughout the world in the context of currently established risk factors.

The most compelling evidence of human carcinogenic risk is revealed through epidemiologic observational studies. The analytic methods of epidemiology are concerned with the formal testing of etiologic hypotheses. The case-control or retrospective method of study is most suitable in studies of rare diseases, in "fishing" for multiple etiologic factors of uncertain significance, and for the initial exploration of a specific etiologic hypothesis. The cohort (prospective, longitudinal, follow-up) study is advantageous in that it provides a direct measure of the incidence or risk of developing a disease in individuals with specified characteristics, and is most suitable for testing a particular hypothesis which has already been developed from prior retrospective or prevalence studies.

Another method of investigation available to the epidemiologist is the randomized clinical trial, wherein the investigator has direct control over the assignment of individuals to study groups. In the context of nutritional intervention or preventive trials, supplementation or modification of dietary intake may serve to inhibit the onset or progression of neoplastic disease in persons at risk.

There are various methodologic approaches that may be employed in developing and testing hypotheses concerning human nutrition and cancer. Hypotheses may be generated based upon studies of average per capita food balance data or surveys of household food inventories. An example used repeatedly in this conference is the correlation among specific countries of average per capita total fat consumption with age-adjusted breast or colon cancer mortality. We recognize that food balance or food disappearance data and surveys of households are limited in that they do not provide an adequate description of the relationship between diet and cancer in individuals.

Dietary data gathered and analyzed at the individual level may use a combination of techniques, such as weighed food records, diaries, recall methods, and food frequencies (number of times a food is consumed per unit of time and average portion sizes of foods consumed). Diet histories are methods for determining usual dietary intake patterns over prolonged periods of time and generally consist of qualitative and quantitative measures of nutrient consumption (Sorenson, 1982).

The major strength of epidemiologic studies is their focus on human populations. They obviate the need for extrapolating from animal data or from extremely high doses to low doses. However, the conduct and interpretation of epidemiologic studies is complicated by inherent variability within and among human populations, changing lifestyle practices and various potential sources of bias in data collection and analysis. Our measurements of dietary and other lifestyle practices need to be tested for their reliability, validity, sensitivity to reveal narrow but biologically significant differences, and to achieve some degree of dose stratification.

Evidence that human exposure to a chemical substance may affect cancer risk may be more readily explored through long-term bioassays in animals and combinations of short-term screening methods for detecting genotoxicity, cell transformation, and modifications of response to chemical, biological, and physical initiators.

Our panel this afternoon will be concerned with the methodologies of risk assessment. In arriving at decisions concerning risk assessment, there are several key questions that need to be addressed:

Who is exposed--proportion of population at risk?

What is the nature and degree of exposure--onset, duration, intensity of exposure?

(The Occupational Safety and Health Administration's minimal criteria for accepting a non-positive result required 20 years of exposure and at least 30 years of observation after initial exposure) (1980)

What excess risk is experienced by the population exposed?

What other exposures need to be considered, that may have provided additive, synergistic, or antagonistic interactions?

The steps involved in the process of risk assessment or risk analysis may be outlined as follows (Rall, 1981):

a) Identification of potential risks--laboratory studies and preliminary epidemiologic studies.

b) Evaluation and quantification of risk--potency of agent = relative risk and dose-response estimation.

c) Assessment of risk within the population--generalizability of research studies.

d) Risk assessment and risk reduction--the social, political, and scientific process of decision-making.

Since it is difficult to determine the "safe" level of human exposure to any suspect carcinogen or co-carcinogen with any degree of confidence, the concepts of "acceptable risk" and "risk-benefit analysis" have emerged in counterpoint to the issue of "zero risk". The Subcommittee on Environmental Carcinogenesis of the National Cancer Advisory Board (1977) summarized the judgmental nature of risk-benefit analysis as follows:

> "In those cases in which a compound has been proved to be carcinogenic remains the decision to what extent the possible risks to man are counterbalanced by the possible social, economic, or medical benefits of that substance. Scientists must play a major role in these decisions by providing and interpreting the available data. The final decision, however, must be made by society at large through informed governmental regulatory and legislative groups."

Department of Labor, Part VII (1980): Occupational Safety & Health Administration. Identification, classification, and regulation of potential occupational carcinogens. Federal Register 45:5001-5296.
Doll R, Peto R (1981): The causes of cancer: Quantitative estimates of avoidable risks of cancer in the United States today. J Natl Cancer Inst 66:1192-1308.
General criteria for assessing the evidence for carcinogenicity of chemical substances. Report of the Sub-committee on Environmental Carcinogenesis. National Cancer Advisory Board (1977). J Natl Cancer Inst 58:461-465.

Rall DP (1981): Issues in the determination of acceptable risk. Ann NY Acad Sci 363:139-144.

Sorenson AW (1982): Assessment of nutrition in epidemiologic studies. IN Schottenfeld D, Fraumeni JF Jr (eds): Cancer Epidemiology and Prevention. Philadelphia: Saunders, pp 434-474.

Wynder EL, Gori GB (1977): Contribution of the environment to cancer incidence. An epidemiologic exercise. J Natl Cancer Inst 58:825-832.

Diet, Nutrition, and Cancer:
From Basic Research to Policy Implications, pages 203–219
© *1983 Alan R. Liss, Inc., 150 Fifth Avenue, New York, NY 10011*

RISK ASSESSMENT OF DIETARY CARCINOGENS AND
TUMOR PROMOTERS

Gary M. Williams
John H. Weisburger
Naylor Dana Institute for Disease Prevention
American Health Foundation
Valhalla, New York 10595-1599

MECHANISMS OF CARCINOGENESIS

Chemical carcinogenesis involves two major processes: the conversion of a normal cell to a neoplastic cell, generally referred to as initiation, and the subsequent progressive growth of the neoplastic cell to form a tumor, which may be described as neoplastic progression.

Carcinogens that initiate the process of neoplastic conversion generally operate at the molecular level as reactive species either in their parent form, or following enzymatic biotransformation to such a species within the host. Considerable evidence, particularly the fact that the neoplastic cell is a permanently altered cell, supports the concept that DNA is a critical target. Therefore, carcinogens with the ability to damage DNA through formation of covalent adducts have been referred to as genotoxic carcinogens (Weisburger and Williams, 1980).

Nongenotoxic chemicals that are active in the subsequent stage of neoplastic progression, such as promoters, can, under specific test conditions, increase the occurrence of neoplasms in experimental animals and thus, are classified as carcinogens. To distinguish this type of carcinogen from the genotoxic type, the term epigenetic has been applied to non-genotoxic agents which enhance oncogenesis through indirect mechanisms (Weisburger and Williams, 1980).

FOODBORNE GENOTOXIC CARCINOGENS

The determination of the genotoxicity of an agent requires evidence of its ability to damage DNA. This can be obtained using a variety of biochemical or physicochemical techniques, but the most expeditious approach is by assay of acitivity in a battery genetic toxicology tests (Williams, 1980a).

The Ames Salmonella mutagenicity test has been extensively utilized for detecting mutagenic materials in food (Haroun and Ames, 1981). The presence of such mutagens is subject for concern, but, since certain of mutagens, such as the flavonoids quercetin and kaempferol, have not been found to be carcinogenic (Morino et al, 1982), it is essential that bacterial mutagenicity data be supported by other evidence before conclusions on hazard are drawn. In this regard, the test developed by Williams and associates (1980b) using freshly isolated hepatocytes to measure DNA repair synthesis as evidence of DNA damage offers some important advantages as an additional assay in a battery of tests.

In the hepatocyte primary culture (HPC)/DNA repair test, the intact hepatocytes, unlike subcellular enzyme systems, provide a balance of biotransformation pathways, including detoxification reactions. In addition, the end point of DNA repair measured in the test is a specific biochemical indicator of genotoxicity.

The HPC/DNA repair test has been effective in detecting a variety of naturally occurring carcinogens including pyrrolizidine alkaloids, which in a specific comparative study were not readily detected in the Ames test (Williams et al, 1980). A significant finding in the HPC/DNA repair test is that the flavonoids quercitin and kaempferol have been inactive (Williams, 1982). An important conclusion stemming from comparison of results in the tests of Ames and Williams is that agents positive in both are almost certainly carcinogenic (Williams, 1982).

Thus, reliable methodologies are available for the identification of genotoxic components of food. A number of naturally occurring carcinogenic substances present in food from microbial or plant sources have been shown to be genotoxic (Williams, 1982). In addition, products formed during cooking have been identified as mutagenic and carcinogenic (Nagao et al, 1980; Shelby and Matusushima, 1981). The pyrolysate product Trp P1 is positive in the HPC/DNA repair test (Williams, 1979) and subsequently was shown to be carcinogenic (Matsukura et al, 1981). IQ,a product formed in fried meat or fish, is also genotoxic (Williams, 1982). IQ is a heterocyclic compound with methyl group ortho to an amino substituent. This structure is similar to experimental carcinogens which produce colon and breast cancer and, therefore, IQ is a candidate for such action.

In studies on dietary sources of gastric carcinogens, Weisburger et al. (1980) found that incubation of fish with nitrite yielded mutagenic activity which subsequently was found to produce stomach cancer in rats.

Clearly, a number of foodborne genotoxins which may be involved in human cancer have been detected.

HEALTH RISK ANALYSIS FOR GENOTOXIC CARCINOGENS

Genotoxic carcinogens have a number of characteristics (Table 1) which must be considered in the analysis of their risk to humans.

Table 1. Properties of Genotoxic Carcinogens

---

1. Occasionally active with single exposure.
2. Frequently active at low (i.e. subtoxic) doses.
3. Can have additive or synergistic effects with one another.
4. Can be active transplacentally and carcinogenicity often increased in neonates.
5. Subcarcinogenic effects can be made manifest by subsequent promoting action.
6. Effects can be enhanced by co-carcinogens.
7. Organotropism shifted by inhibitors of biotransformation.

The underlying action of genotoxic carcinogens with DNA is at least theoretically a process that could occur at low levels of exposure. Consequently, it has been suggested that there would be no threshold for the carcinogenicity of chemicals. Experimental proof of this, however, is deficient.

Relatively few detailed dose-response studies with diverse chemical carcinogens have been reported and all of these involve genotoxic carcinogens. The classic study of Bryan and Shimkin (1943) has been utilized by mathematical statisticians to formulate the theoretical shape of dose-response curves, especially in extrapolations to low level effects. In this study, mice were given subcutaneous injections of three polycyclic aromatic hydrocarbons and the evaluation was based on the occurrence of sarcomas at the site of injection. With all three hydrocarbons, the dose-response curves assumed an S-shaped pattern typically seen in virtually all pharmacological dose-response studies and from which it is possible to determine a no-effect level. Indeed, the actual data in the report by Bryan and Shimkin show that with the three carcinogens there were several doses at the low end which yielded no increase in tumors. Nonetheless, because of the possible errors involved and the relatively small number of animals used, mathematical theory has been invoked to suggest that the overall response might involve a one-hit linear model with no threshold (Mantel and Bryan, 1961). Over the last 30 years, this experiment has been interpreted in a number of different ways, although the mathematical formulation and approach developed by Cornfield (1977) seems to approximate the actual experimental values best. The analysis of Cornfield reveals that even if carcinogenesis is a one-hit phenomenon, the existence of a threshold is not precluded.

Druckrey's group (Druckrey, 1967) in Germany has contributed dose-response studies, performed under exacting identical conditions, with a number of chemical carcinogens belonging to the class of aromatic amines and azo dyes and also with diethylnitrosamine. The interpretation of these studies involving cancer induction in several sites has been that with these very powerful carcinogens the overall yield of cancer is proportional to the total dose administered but that the latent period to disease is a function of the dose rate. Druckrey has further interpreted the results as signifying the absence of a threshold and suggested that an apparent threshold was present only because of the limitation of lifespan (900-1000 days) under the conditions of the experiment.

In the large-scale study conducted by the U.S. National Center for Toxicological Research involving dosages randing from 150 ppm down to 30 ppm of N-2-fluorenylacetamide, fed to mice, two organs were affected, the urinary bladder and the liver (Symposium, 1981). For tumors in the urinary bladder, a definite no-effect level was found in this experiment conducted for 33 months, an extraordinarily long-time. However, for liver tumors, especially for the groups of animals that remained alive through 33 months, a straight line response was calculated from 150-30 ppm. It was further suggested that this response corresponded to a linear model going through zero. The experimental design aimed for a 1% response and for that reason large numbers of animals were used at levels of 30, 40, and 45 ppm, and, as might be expected, the complex biological response did not differ for such closely spaced doses. An intriguing question is what the response might have been if the spacing of doses at the lower end were wider and went, for example, to 3 or even 1 ppm. It is possible that such levels of this powerful carcinogen affecting several target organs would have shown no appreciable effect even in large samples. Such exposure levels to this chemical would have been readily measurable chemically and correspond to levels of environmental carcinogens which have been the subject of concern.

Thus, experimental dose-response studies with genotoxic carcinogens have clearly revealed activity at low doses, but some evidence of threshold effects even with very potent carcinogens such as polycyclic aromatic hydrocarbons, aromatic amines and nitrosamines.

The potential for a threshold is even more likely with certain other genotoxic carcinogens. Animal experiments performed under similar conditions reveal that in contrast to the high incidence of hepatocellular carcinoma in rats in less than a year produced by dietary intake of 100 ppb of aflatoxin B_1 (and indeed this chemical can induce liver cancer at levels as low as 1 ppb), safrole at dietary levels of 5000 ppm produces liver cancer in lower yield and after a longer latent period. This is a difference in of almost 100,000-fold higher levels of safrole compared to aflatoxin perhaps owing to the distinct pathways of metabolic activation (Weisburger and Williams, 1982a); only a small fraction of safrole is converted to the ultimate carcinogenic form, whereas with aflatoxin the required epoxidation of the molecule may occur to a much greater extent. These observations suggest that for procarcinogens which require metabolic activation and undergo detoxification, biotransformation processes may render low doses ineffective (Weisburger and Williams, 1982a). Moreover, the reactive electrophile, the ultimate carcinogen, can undergo reactions with non-specific cellular nucleophiles and, thus, not reach cirtical targets. Even DNA itself or the chromosomal apparatus as a whole may not uniformly react at significant points with regard to cancer induction. Thus, from the point of view of the long sequence, starting with administration of a procarcinogen leading to the specific cancer-inducing molecular interaction, there are many non-productive side reactions which may result in threshold no-effect levels with genotoxic agents at very low dosages.

Nevertheless, the properties of genotoxic carcinogens (Table 1) dictate that it is essential to minimize human exposure to these agents. In particular, conditions of increased susceptibility, possible additive effects and the potential of sitations leading to tumor enhancement unpredictably increase their risk. Therefore, at present, genotoxic carcinogens should be regarded as qualitative hazards and their exposure to humans reduced as much as practical (Weisburger and Williams, 1981a).

Methods are available to establish whether or not a given substance is genotoxic (Weisburger and Williams, 1981b). If it is, rational decisions can be made as to the kind of additional data needed to evaluate the nature of the risk of the presence of such agents in the human environment. Some of the elements that can be useful for such a risk evaluation are shown in Table 2.

Table 2. Data Points for Consideration in Risk Analysis of Genotoxic Carcinogens

---

1. Species/strain/organs affected.
2. Dose-response characteristics for each organ affected.
3. Characteristics of biotransformation — ratio detoxification/activation.
4. Nature of human exposure — period of life, level, duration, etc.
5. Probability of exposure to other genotoxins or enhancers of carcinogenesis.

Quantitative carcinogenesis studies make it possible to evaluate the strength of the expresseion of any genotoxic effect or relative to that of other genotoxic carcinogens. In a species to species comparison of carcinogenicity, Williams et al (1978) found for six selected carcinogens that therewas an animal system as sensitive or more sensitive than humans. Thus, delineation of dose characteristics in the most sensitive species would permit a conservative linear extrapolation to low doses that would not represent a significant human hazard, providing contrary indications from the other data points are not present. Thus, although there is no simple procedure for using the data points recommended, they provide a guide to the kind of information necessary to formulating acceptable exposures in situations where it is not practical to completely eliminate a genotoxin form the human environment.

FOODBORNE TUMOR PROMOTERS

Chemicals that facilitate the progression of initiated or altered cells to tumor formation will function operationally as carcinogens in situations in which pre-existing abnormal cells are present. Consequently, agents of this type have been categorized as epigenetic carcinogens. The designation of such agents as epigenetic depends firstly upon a reliable demonstration of lack of genotoxicity. Secondly, the agents should display some other biological effect which could account for their production of tumors under specific conditions. An important class of carcinogens which are not genotoxic is that which mechanistic studies have revealed to have the property of tumor promoters or enhancers.

The promoting activity of materials that have been demonstrated to be nongenotoxic can be definitely established in in vivo systems by the demonstration of an enhancing effect on tumorigenesis when the materials are administered after, but not before a genotoxic carcinogen. The most extensive study of structural requirements for promotion has been done with phorbol compounds which are skin tumor promoters. In addition, there are reliable in vivo models for tumor promotion in a variety of other organs including liver, mammary gland, bladder and intestine, among others (Slaga et al, 1978).

Recently, attempts have been made to develop in vitro systems for detection of tumor promoters (see Heidelberger et al and Weinstein et al in Slaga et al, 1978). Recently, Yotti et al (1979) and Murray and Fitzgerald (1979) independently reported that phorbol esters inhibited intercellular communication between cultured cells. Subsequently, this effect has been demonstrated for a variety of promoters (Trosko et al, 1981) and extended to other cell systems such as liver cultures (Williams, 1980a; 1981). Evidence suggests that the latency of initiated cells may be due to regulatory restraint imposed by surrounding normal cells through intercellular communication mediated by gap junctions. Thus, the endpoint of inhibition of intercellular communication, in addition to its demonstrated sensitivity for promoting agents, has the advantage of being possibly related to a critical effect of certain types of promoters in vivo.

Thus, a variety approaches are available to identify food-borne materials with promoting action. Foodborne agents that act as tumor promoters include contaminants such as DDT and diethylstilbestrol and additives such as saccharin (Williams, 1982). Also, the essential amino acid tryptophan, probably through an as yet unknown metabolite(s), can act a promoter of bladder carcinogenesis. The phorbol esters which are naturally-occurring substances derived from the plant Croton tiglium L are effective skin tumor promoters and recently another naturally occurring skin tumor promoter, teleocidin B, was identified (Fujiki et al, 1979).

Dietary fat has been established to produce a produce a promoting action in colon carcinogenesis through enhancement of secretion of bile acids (Narisawa et al, 1974; Chomchai et al, 1974) and in breast cancer probably through increased elaboration of pituitary hormones (Carrol, 1975; Chan and Cohen, 1975). Fat and other dietary components through their modulating effects on carcinogenesis are suspected to play a determining role in several major human cancers.

RISK ASSESSMENT OF TUMOR PROMOTERS

The concept of promotion in chemical carcinogenesis is almost 50 years old. However, the focus of many of the

early studies was on the mechanism of action of the mouse
skin tumor promoters, croton oil and of phorbol esters
(Slaga et al, 1978) and thus many of the concepts on the
phenomenon of promotion are based on mouse skin studies.
The identification of cellular receptors for phorbol esters
indicates that this kind of promoter may operate by specific
mechanisms not necessarily pertaining to other agents such
as saccharin or bile acids, or certain of the chlorinated
hydrocarbons such as DDT. The accumulated information on
the properties of tumor promoters (Table 3), nevertheless
indicates that their effects differ significantly from those
of genotoxic carcinogens.

Table 3. Properties of Promoters

---

1. Not demonstrated to be active with single exposure.
2. May be active at low dose, but require a level of
    exposure to produce relevant biological effect.
3. Additivity uncertain. Can inhibit one another.
4. Only DES active transplacentally.
5. No evidence of enhanced susceptibility of neonates.
6. Shifts in organotropism not reported.

Phorbol esters are active as promoters at low doses,
but unfortunately there are few quantitative data on the
effects of other promoting agents. Thus, there have not
been many carefully conducted dose-response studies or
investigations dealing with the functioning of such agents.
Of great relevance and practical importance, are studies on
the precise mechanism of action for each kind of promoter as
regards the specific molecular events in the organ
affected. Information of this type is needed for hormones
with effects on the endocrine system, bile acids as they
affect the intestinal tract, or pesticides, drugs,
artificial sweeteners or even the essential amino acid
L-tryptophan, as they might affect certain other organs such
as the liver or the urinary bladder.

Where dose-response studies involving promoting agents have been done, it was usually in the context of a carcinogen bioassay with limited dose levels and dose ranges. Under these conditions, it was apparent, however, that activity was seen mainly at very high dose levels with a sharp drop-off occurring as doses were lowered even relatively slightly. Such findings were made for the production of rat bladder tumors by saccharin, and mouse liver tumors by chlorinated hydrocarbons. It will be important to further delineate such effects of dose on response in specifically designed experiments with a genotoxic initiator, and the promoter or epigenetic agent given at a number of dose levels including one or two in the range of practical exposure.

In the case of saccharin, a beginning has been made to delineate a dose-response curve for urinary bladder carcinogenesis. In a model study, Cohen et al. (1979) have demonstrated that saccharin, given after a bladder carcinogen, can act as a promoter at 5% (50,000 ppm) in the diet. Likewise, intake of only 2% L-tryptophan had a similar affect suggesting that this amino acid (or metabolites) is a stronger promoter. Utilizing a different carcinogen, Nakanishi et al (1980) delineated a dose-response curve for production of bladder hyperplasia by saccharin. It was found that for male and female rats levels lower than 10,000 ppm, or 1% in the diet had no effect. Likewise, epidemiological studies have failed to demonstrate any effect of saccharin use in humans, especially when corrected for confounding factors such as cigarette smoking (Wynder and Stellman, 1980). This finding is perhaps not unexpected considering human use levels in relation to the high levels that are necessary for producing promoting effects in the animal models.

Hormones, especially estrogens, have been classified as promoters as well. A study by Highman et al (1977) shows that, in mice bearing the mammary tumor virus, which acts as the genotoxic event to yield cancers, DES and also interestingly equi-estrogenic amounts of the naturally-occurring estradiol had a dose-related effect in mammary carcinogenesis. Of great importance in the light of the concepts discussed, is the fact that in mice free of MTV, and thus presumably endowed with mammary gland cells containing a normal genetic structure, DES levels up to 500 ppb did not produce mammary carcinogenesis. This study illustrates the point that in order to produce tumors, promoters require a specific antecedent gene change which can be mediated by an appropriate genotoxic reactant which can be chemical, viral, or physical (radiation) or can arise from inherited genetic abnormalities.

Current evidence suggest that a number of hepatocarcinogens such as phenobarbital, tetrachlorethane, and above all DDT, are not genotoxic carcinogens but can act as liver tumor promoters (Williams, 1981). There is virtually no reliable information as to dose response with these chlorinated hydrocarbons studied as promoters. A study by Peraino et al. (1980) of liver tumor promotion by phenobarbital revealed a broad dose response from 0.010 ppm to 0.250 ppm. The lowest dose 0.002 ppm had no effect on the incidence of rats with liver tumors, but did slightly increase the multiplicity of tumors. Detailed epidemiological studies have revealed no evidence at this time that any of these chemicals have had an effect in enhancing human tumor formation in people occupationally or environmentally exposed to chemicals such as DDT or other organochlorine compounds (Hayes et al, 1971; Deichmann and MacDonald, 1977) or given phenobarbital as a medication (Clemmenson and Hjalgrim-Jensen, 1978).

Thus, the knowledge of the actions of tumor promoters indicates that a number of elements must be considered in formulating a risk analysis (Table 4).

Table 4. Data Points for Consideration in Risk Analysis of Tumor Promoters

---

1. Species/strain/organ affected.
2. Dose-response characteristics.
3. Biological effects at promoting doses that underly activity and liklihood of similar effect in humans.
4. Pharmacokinetics in susceptible species compared to humans.
5. Nature of human exposure, intermittent versus continuous.
6. Probability of prior genotoxin exposures or presence of initiated cells in potential human target organ.

As with genotoxic carcinogens generally applicable quantitative procedures are not yet available, but evaluation of essential data can be employed in a realistic risk asessment. For example, in the instance of colon cancer where bile acids and bile acid concentrations appear to be the relevant measures of promoting stimuli, reduction of the concentration of total bile acids in the intestine by only about 50%, either by lowering the intake of total dietary fat or by increasing the amount of dietary cereal fiber which increases stool bulk, converts a high risk situation to one of lowered risk (Reddy et al, 1980).

CONCLUSIONS

The developments presented in this paper clearly suggest that the health risk analysis for promoters needs to be different from that applying to genotoxic carcinogens. Some of the elements we visualize as bearing on health risk analysis, with respect to genotoxic carcinogens and the distinct data points required for nongenotoxic promoters, are listed in tables 2 and 4.

The history of carcinogenesis provides a number of instances where, under conditions of occupational or therapeutic exposure, genotoxic carcinogens have induced cancer in humans. In the context of environmental agents that can act either as genotoxic carcinogens or as nongenotoxic modifers, namely co-carcinogens or tumor promoters, we have classified a number of such agents as they relate to the main human cancers in the North American population (Weisburger and Williams, 1982b). Our conclusion is that approximately 40-60% of cancer is due to lifestyle factos, of which nutrition play a major role (Williams et al, 1982). In addition, in other parts of the world, such as the African and Asian continents, genotoxic agents such as those produced by molds or plants in the form of mycotoxins or pyrrolizidine alkaloids appear to be involved.

A clear distinction can be made in the broad area of nutritional carcinogenesis as related to large bowel cancer between the risk analysis applicable to genotoxic carcinogens and those agents that play a major promoting role. For the promoters, in this instance bile acids present in the intestine, it has been shown that reduction of the concentration of bile acids, either by a lower intake of dietary fat or by an increased intake of bulk produced by cereal fiber, significantly lowers the cancer incidence. This is supported by comparison of the high incidence of colon cancer in the western world to that in Japan (modulator: fat level) or to that in Finland (modulator: colon dietary fiber level). In these cases, the applicable bile acid concentrations go from 11.7 mg/g total bile acids in subjects living in the New York metropolitan area to about 4 mg/g total bile acids for Japanese subjects or 4.6 mg/g for Finish subjects. Thus, a reduction by a factor of only about 3 changes, a highly effective promoting level to one that is weak. In animal studies, similar findings have been made. Indeed, in one experiment groups of animals were given identical initiating genotoxic carcinogen delivered to the colonic mucosa. In the group of animals where the promoting stimulus was totally removed by removing the luminal flow of bile acids and other intestinal elements by a colostomy no cancers at all were found Narisawa et al, 1978).

It seems useful, therefore, in current and future activities in health risk analysis to delineate as a first important step using the appropriate contemporary tests, the question whether a given product is genotoxic. If it is, and human exposure cannot be eliminated, appropriate dose-response studies need to be devised, using several species and in the light of the information from metabolism and pharmacokinetics through which the complexities of metabolic activation and detoxification can be elucidated. A series of data points permit reasonable conclusions to be drawn regarding health risk.

If appropriate tests for genotoxicity suggest that a material is negative, an appropriate series of tests would include the determination of the possible promoting effects at specific target organs. This, in turn, permits the development of a protocol involving a suitable genotoxic initiating carcinogen given at a dose level such that the promoting action of the unknown agent can be studied. This test series should provide a basis for the determination of a no-effect level and in a more elaborate series of tests the possible reversibility of the effect. In addition, information needs to be developed on the metabolism and biological effects which underlie the action of the agent. In all these instances, dose response studies should necessarily include dosages approximating the maximum expected human exposure. The combined information may lead to determination of safe human exposure levels.

The process of risk assessment is clearly complex and must be performed in a flexible manner for each individual element in the human environment. With increasing knowledge of mechanisms of action and properties of different types of agents involved in the carcinogenic process, the prospect is bright that factors relating to human cancer, in particular those contributed by diet, can be controlled.

REFERENCES

Bryan WR, Shimkin MB (1943). Quantitative analysis of dose-response data obtained with three carcinogenic hydrocarbons in strain C3H male mice. J Natl Cancer Inst 3:503.

Carroll KK (1975). Experimental evidence of dietary factors and hormone-dependent cancers. Cancer Res 35:3374.

Chan PC, Cohen LA (1975). Dietary fat and growth promotion of rat mammary tumor. Cancer Res 35:3384.

Chomchai C, Bhadrachari N, Nigro ND (1974). The effect of bile on the induction of experimental intestinal tumors in rats. Dis Colon Rectum 17:310.

Clemmesen J, Hjalgrim-Jensen S (1978). Is phenobarbital carcinogenic? A follow-up of 8078 epileptics. Ecotox and Environ Safety 1:457.

Cornfield J (1977). Carcinogenic risk assessment. Science 198:693.

Cohen SM, Arai M, Jacobs JB, Friedell GH (1979). Promoting effect of saccharin and DL-tryptophan in urinary bladder carcinogenesis. Cancer Res 39:1207.

Deichmann WB, MacDonald WE (1977). Organo-chlorine pesticides and liver cancer deaths in the United States, 1930-1972. Ecotoxicol Environ Safety 1:89.

Druckrey H (1967). Quantitative aspects in chemical carcinogenesis. In Potential Carcinogenic Hazards from Drugs. Truhaut R (ed): Berlin: Springer-Verlag, p 60.

Fujiki H, Mori Masami M, Nakayasu M, Terada M, Sugimura T (1979).A possible naturally occurring tumor promoter, teleocidin B from streptomyces. Biochem Biophys Res Comm 90:976.

Haroun L, Ames BN (1981). The Salmonella mutagenicity test: An overview. In Stich HF, San RHC (eds): "Short-term Tests for Chemical Carcinogens," New York: Sringer-Verlag, p 108.

Hayes WJ, Dale WE, Pizkle CI (1971). Evidenceof safety of longterm, high, oral doses of DDT for man. Arch Environ Health 22:119.

Highman B, Norvell MJ, Shellenberger TE (1977). Pathological changes in female C3H mice continuously fed diets containing diethylstilbestrol or 17β–estradiol. J Environ Pathol Toxicol 1:1.

Murray AW, Fitzgerald DJ (1979). Tumor promoters inhibit metabolic cooperation in cocultures of epidermal and 3T3 cells. Biochem Biophys Res Commun 91:395.

Matsukura N, Kawachi T, Morino K, Ohgaki H, Sugimura, T (1981). Carcinogenicity in mice of mutagenic compounds from a tryptophan pyrolyzate. Science 213:346.

Mantel N, Bryan WR (1961). Safety testing of carcinogenic agents. J Natl Cancer Inst 27:455.

Morino K, Matsukura N, Kawachi T, Ohgaki H, Sugimura T and Hirono I (1982). Carcinogenicity test of quercitin and rutin in golden hamsters by oral administration. Carcinogenesis 3:93.

Narisawa T, Magadia NE, Weisburger JH, Wynder EL (1974). Promoting effect of bile acilds on colon carcinogenesis after intrarectal instillation of N–methyl–N'–nitro–N–nitrosogianidine in rats. J Natl Cancer Inst 55:1093.

Narisawa T, Reddy BS, Weisburger JH (1978). Effect of bile acids and dietary fat on large bowel carcinogenesis in animal models. Gastroenterol Jpn 13:206.

Nagao M, Takahashi Y, Yahagi T, Sugimura T, Takeda K, Shudo K, Okamoto T (1980). Mutagenicities of γ–carboline derivatives related to potent mutagens found in tryptophan pyrolysates. Carcinogenesis 1:451.

Nakanishi K, Hagiwara A, Shibata M, Imaida K, Tatematsu M, Ito N (1980). Dose–response of saccharin in the induction of urinary bladder lesions in rats pretreated with N–butyl–N–(4–hydroxybutyl)nitrosamine. J Natl Cancer Inst 65:1005.

Peraino C, Staffeldt EF, Haugen DA, Lombard LS, Stevens FJ, Fry RJM (1980). Effects of varying the dietary concentration of phenobarbital on its enhancement of 2-Acetylaminofluorene–induced hepatic tumorigenesis. Cancer Res 40:3268.

Reddy BS, Cohen LA, McCoy GD, Hill P, WeisburgerJH, Wynder EL (1980). Nutrition and its relationship to cancer. Adv Cancer Res 32:237.

Shelby MD, Matsushima T (1981). Mutagens and carcinogens in the diet and digestive tract. Mutation Res 85:177.

Slaga TJ, Sivak A, Boutwell RK (1978). "Carcinogenesis A Comprehensive Survey." New York: Raven Press.

Symposium (1981). Re-examination of the ED_{01} study. Overview. Fund Appl Toxicol 1: 28-128.

Trosko JE, Yotti LP, Dawson B, Chang CC (1981). In vitro assay for tumor promoters. In Stich HF, San RHC (eds): "Short-Term tests for Chemical Carcinogens," New York: Springer-Verlag, p 420.

Weisburger JH, Marquardt H, Hirota N, Mori H, Williams GM,(1980). Induction of glandular stomach cancer in rats with an extract of nitrite-treated fish. J Natl Cancer Inst 64:163.

Weisburger JH, Williams GM (1980). Chemical Carcinogens In Doull J, Klaasen CD, Amdur MO (eds): "Toxicology the Basic Science of Poisons," New York: Macmillan Publishing, p 84.

Weisburger JH, Williams GM (1981a). Basic requirements for health risk analysis: The decision point approach for systematic carcinogen testing. In Richmond CR, Walsh PJ Copenhaver ED (eds): "Health Risk Analysis," Philadelphia: Franklin Institute Press, p 249.

Weisburger JH, Williams GM (1981b). Carcinogen testing: Current problems and new approaches. Science 214:401.

Weisburger JM, Williams GM (1982a). Metabolism of chemical carcinogens. In Becker FF (ed): "Cancer: A Comprehensive Treatise," New York: Plenum Publishing Company, p 241.

Weisburger JH, Williams GM (1982b). Chemical Carcinogenesis. In Holland JF, Frei E III (eds): "Cancer Medicine,"Philadelphia: Lea and Febiger, p 42.

Williams GM (1979). Liver cell culture systems for the study of hepatocarcinogenesis. In Margison GP (ed): "Advances in Medical Onclogy, Research and Education, Proceedings of the XIIth International Cancer Congress,"New York: Pergamon Press, p 273.

Williams GM (1980a). Classification of genotoxic and epigenetic hepatocarcinogens using liver culture assays. Ann N Y Acad Sci 349:273.

Williams GM (1980b). The detection of chemical mutagens by DNA repair and mutagenesis in liver cultures. In de Serres FJ, Hollaender A (eds): "Chemical Mutagens," New York: Plenum Press, p 61.

Williams GM (1981). Liver carcinogenesis: The role for some chemicals of an epigenetic mechanism of liver-tumour promotion involving modification of the cell membrane. Fd Cosmet Toxicol 19:577.

Williams GM (1982) Mechanisms of action of foodborne carcinogens. Proceedings Environmental Aspects of Cancer; the Role of Macro and Micro Components of Food, Livingston GE, Leveille GA, Weisburger JH (eds) Food and Nutrition Press, in press.

Williams GM, Mori H, Hirono I, Nagao M (1980). Genotoxicity of pyrrolizidine alkaloids in the hepatocyte primary culture/DNA repair test. Mutation Res 79:1.

Williams BM, Leff A, Weisburger JH (1978). A species to species comparison of carcinogenicity data, with human extrapolation. Final Report NIEHS Contract ES-6-2130. Research Triangle Park: National Institute of Environmental Health Sciences.

Williams GM, Weisburger JH, Wynder EL (1982). Lifestyle and cancer etiology. In Stich H (ed): "Carcinogens and Mutagens in the Environment," Boca Raton: CRC Press, in press.

Wynder EL, Stellman SD (1980). Bladder-cancer and artificial sweeteners: a methodological issue. Science 210:447.

Yotti LP, Chang CC, Trosko JE (1979). Elimination of metabolic cooperation in Chinese hamster cells by a tumor promoter. Science 206:1089.

Diet, Nutrition, and Cancer:
From Basic Research to Policy Implications, pages 221–239
© *1983 Alan R. Liss, Inc., 150 Fifth Avenue, New York, NY 10011*

MOUSE + MAN + MATHEMATICS = MEANING OR MESS?

Marvin A. Schneiderman

Clement Associates, Inc.
Arlington, Virginia

RISK ASSESSMENT AND SOME CURRENT PROBLEMS

Risk assessment is a relatively new tool that should
help improve human health. Well and thoughtfully done,
it can help man in his humanness to do things that preserve
the species. As Lord Ashby has pointed out, man can deliberately change his future, and need not, like other animals
be merely a reactor to unanticipated hazards and dangers
(Ashby 1978). This should have some survival advantages.
In a society in which there is an awareness of dangers,
risk analysis can help direct our efforts toward reducing
the greatest of those dangers, or the most frightening
of the dangers, or the most easily modified of those dangers.
We must recognize, however, that risk assessment is not
essential to reducing dangers--but perhaps it can help
us move in a generally rational and reasonable way.

The most frightening of the dangers to many people
is the prospect of developing cancer. It is sufficiently
frightening that recognizing cigarette smoking as a major
cause of cancer, lots of people have stopped smoking cigarettes, and cigarette manufacturers today are making cigarettes with half the tars of the cigarettes of 20 years
ago (U.S. Department of Health and Human Services 1982).
Substantial research resources are devoted to uncovering
causes, and/or possible preventers of cancer. Having still
not prevented as much cancer by these means as we would
like, we have become concerned that aspects of where we
live, what we drink and what we eat (or don't eat), may
have something to do with our later developing cancer.

Our anticancer efforts grow greater as our population grows older. In the United States, more than half of all cancers (in 1979, 61.5%) occur in persons 65 or over (U.S. National Center for Health Statistics 1982). Some of us are concerned because we see cancer falling disproportionately more heavily on some subsections of the population. This concern arises not out of some false egalitarian desire that everyone be equally burdened, but rather from a desire that the sources of burden be better understood--so that the burden might be lightened for all persons.

Richard Peto, at this conference indicated that one of our aims should be to avert disasters. With respect to cancer he has identified at least two disaster causes-- cigarette smoking and exposure to asbestos. The recent (last 50 years, perhaps) history of cancer research has taken on some aspects of this disaster avoidance approach-- mostly in the search for carcinogens--things that of them- selves cause cancer. Only in the very recent past has substantial consideration been given to things, or behavior, or interactions that might prevent cancer, the multistage theories of the process involved in the development of cancer not withstanding (Armitage, Doll 1961). The multi- stage process sees cancer as developing through a series of steps, the earliest of which starts the process and is thus called initiation (and the starters are called initiators), and the last of which, which is called promo- tion, brings the process into observable form (Day, Brown 1980). With respect to diet and cancer, I see disaster avoidance taking two quite different directions. Historic- ally, people have looked for excesses--exposure in the food we eat to things that "cause" cancer. On the other hand, some other researchers have been looking for deficien- cies in our diets of things that might prevent cancer. The fact that much cancer seems, within our society at least, to occur in poorer people has been variously ascribed to poor diet (both eating things that shouldn't be eaten, e.g., fats, lots of calories, too much salt or salt-preserved foods, and not eating things that should be, e.g., vitamin C, vitamin A or its precursors, perhaps selenium and some other trace metals), to poor environment, to bad personal habits (cigarette smoking, or having children young, which is related to increased cervical cancer and reduced breast cancer), to living in inner cities, to poorer education-- leading to poorer health habits, etc. (U.S. Department of Health and Human Services 1982; Smith, Smyth 1972; Knowles

1977; Wildavsky 1977; Lambert et al. 1982; Kegeles 1976;
Berg et al. 1977; Higginson 1980; Doll, Peto 1981; Fox,
Adelstein 1978; Higginson, Muir 1979). These things are
sometimes all lumped together and called "life style."
The obvious conclusion is that rich life style is better
than poor life style. (I can just hear some cynical taxpayer
saying, "Is that what we put all that money into research
for, so that you scientists would tell us the obvious?")

With respect to the diet issue, it seems to me that
we've almost returned to the Greeks and the search for
the golden mean. Too much is more than enough, and too
little is not too good either. Stomach cancer is high in
parts of the world where a great proportion of the calories
come from cheap food such as grains, starches, potatoes
(Segi et al. 1969, National Research Council 1982). Breast
cancer and colon cancer are high where a small proportion
of the calories come from grains and starches (Armstrong,
Doll 1975; Segi et al. 1969; Wynder, Mabuchi 1972). Stomach
cancer seems to be "set" (with a propensity established)
by adolescence, if the migrant studies are to be believed
(Haenszel 1961; Haenszel, Correa 1975). This would seem
to indicate that some aspects of diet must be acting as
initiators. Examination of NCI's cancer maps have led
to the hypothesis that colon and rectum cancer might be
modified by migration (to Florida's West Coast, for example)
late in life (Ziegler et al. 1981). That would seem to
indicate that some aspect of the environment, and here,
diet is the most likely candidate, acts like a promoter.

This all brings me back to risk assessment. If we
are to have appropriate (and roughly correct) risk assessments, they have to be based on appropriate and roughly
correct models of the cancer process. If diet, a very
gross catch-all, having only slightly more specificity
that "environment" or "life style" enters into the cancer
process we must construct models of this process (these
processes?) that adequately reflect the impact of diet.
I don't think we've yet done this. The most sophisticated
risk assessment models we have are not sophisticated enough.
I shall return to this.

DISASTER AVOIDANCE: HOW DO WE LEARN WHAT TO AVOID?

If we think of the two causes of cancer disaster (Peto

1982), exposure to cigarette smoke and exposure to asbestos, we see that they are both man-manipulated external causes. Much of cancer research since the second decade of this century, when the first external "cause" was demonstrated in animals, has been directed toward finding external causes similar to cigarette smoke, or asbestos. The major tools for finding these external causes have been long term animal studies. Cancer appears to be similar in all mammals--with some differences in sensitivity, but substantial similarity in the process (Interagency Regulatory Liaison Group 1979). The major animals that have been used are the small rodents which are relatively cheap, easy to handle, and to breed. They have a short life span and thus can be treated for a lifetime. With one or two exceptions, all the materials which have been shown to cause cancer in man have caused cancer in some animal species--usually the rodent. The question of course remains, how good a predicter for humans is the laboratory animal? If the laboratory animal over-predicts--says more things are likely to cause cancer in man than really do, we will have false positives with likely adverse economic consequences for the producer and industrial user of the material. This kind of error has been called "producer risk" (Shewhart 1931). If the laboratory animal under-predicts--says something is OK when it really is a carcinogen--then we have false negatives with likely adverse health consequences to persons exposed to the materials. This kind of error is called "consumer risk."

The animal models have been challenged as imperfect predictors--often with the suggestion that they are too sensitive, predicting too much, leading to false positives, leading to bad economic consequences. Some of the arguments are these: (1) the mouse and rat liver tumors are not "real" predictors of cancer in man. Man has evolved as an animal putting a lot of pressure on his liver (i.e., deliberately drinking fermented and other toxin-containing materials that the liver must detoxify.) Through evolution man has developed a very tough liver. Specially bred mice and rats are not nearly so tough. (2) The lung adenomas in the strain A mouse are not indicative of what might happen to man. This mouse is also too sensitive. (3) The pituitary tumors in some strains of rats are so common (and so uncommon in humans) that they should be disregarded. So should other common "background tumors." (4) The labora-tory animals are too sensitive (or, sometimes, not sensitive enough) to indicate what would happen to humans. (5) Oxygen

tension is high in humans and low in rodents and oxygen tension may play a role in producing cancer. And so on (Gori
1980; Handler 1979).

Given these arguments about the inappropriateness
of the laboratory animal model, there has developed pressure
to pay more attention to human studies. The argument is
made that most materials shown to be carcinogenic in any
species were first shown to be carcinogenic in humans,
anyway. And that goes for both disasters Peto mentioned--
cigarette smoking and asbestos (Calfornia Health and Welfare
Agency 1982). But if we are to avert disasters, we have
to find out about disaster-causers before people have been
exposed to them--not after. Of course, finding out at
anytime serves to reduce the potential for continuing future
disaster. In this light it is worth noting that the Mt. Sinai
group--who have been among the leaders in the study of
workplace exposures to asbestos, have changed their estimates
of the annual number of cancer deaths related to industrial
exposure to asbestos from 50,000 (made in the late 70's)
to 8 to 10 thousand (Nicholson et al. 1981). Whether this
changed estimate is related solely to the fact that asbestos
exposures have been substantially reduced since the first
standards went into effect in 1968 and then made progressively more stringent, is not at all clear. I think other
changes in estimates of intensity of exposure and numbers
exposed have also entered into the estimates.

I believe that the expected future cigarette-related
cancer deaths should probably also be recomputed (downward)
at this time. Proportionately fewer adults are now smoking
than at anytime in the last several decades, although smokers
now smoke more cigarettes. Cigarettes now contain less
tars than did earlier cigarettes (U.S. Department of Health
and Human Services 1982). In the older age groups, which
are now making up proportionately more of the total population and in which the cancer rates are highest, there are
relatively fewer persons who are or ever were cigarette
smokers. (One reason is that cigarette smokers die at
younger ages than non-smokers.) My most recent estimate
is that roughly just under 30% of all newly diagnosed male
cancers, and 10% of new cancers in women are currently
related to cigarette smoking (Davis et al. 1981). I expect
the proportion in women to increase in the remainder of
the century, and the proportion in men to decrease--and
then both to decrease. I write this with some trepidation,

because I've been expecting the proportion to decrease in
males for at least the last ten years--in view of the reduced
proportion of continuing smokers (and the increase portion
of stopped smokers) and the reduced tars in cigarettes--
but this has not yet happened. My mathematical modelling
has probably been too unsophisticated.

Some of the other difficulties in relying on epidemiologic studies reflect the complex world we live in. People
are exposed to many things--making it almost impossible
to pin-point single "causes." Cancer generally has a long
latent period--during which time many other events occur.
Most epidemiologic studies have low power (cancer, despite
its being the second leading cause of death is nonetheless
a rare disease). Finally, for almost every epidemiologic
study that says "Yes, there is an association," there seems
to be another study that says, "We didn't find anything,
here." Peto pointed this out in his review of the vitamin A
and cancer studies (Peto 1982).

In the last decade there have been developed new testing techniques that don't take as long or cost as much as
the animal studies, and that may be predictive (more predictive?) of what will happen to man. These are the so called
short term studies, usually in bacteria, or other cells,
and most often of mutagenesis, rather than carcinogenesis.
They lead to the interesting paradox that on one hand greater
reliance may now be given to the effects in organisms very
far removed from man, while criticism is made of studies on
rodents, as not being fully indicative of what is likely to
happen to man -- rodents being not sufficiently like man.
Surely a mammal is closer to a human than is a salmonella
cell. For example, Robert Squire, in suggesting a scheme
for establishing priorities for preventive or regulatory
action for potential carcinogens (i.e., priorities for
avoiding disaster) allots 25 points to the demonstration
that a material is mutagenic (genotoxic) and 15 points to
the (replicated) demonstration that it is carcinogenic in
two or more independent animal tests (Squire 1981). Thus,
in looking for an objective procedure on which to base
action, Squire gives 67% more weight to a non-carcinogenic
response to lower organisms than to a carcinogenic response
in higher organisms. That this may be intuitively offensive
doesn't make it wrong, however. Think of the demonstration
of the gravitational effects on the speed of fall of light
and heavy bodies.

The study of mutagenesis, and similar carcinogenesis-like action in the short term tests (and lower biological forms) has led several persons, including Dr. Williams to suggest different systems for establishing standards for materials identified as genotoxic and materials identified as not genotoxic (Williams 1982). At present, so far as I know, there are no agreed upon standards for identifying a material as clearly non-genotoxic (or as genotoxic). Lave et al., in their attempt to find a battery of short term tests with minimum error, accepted one positive test as enough to label a material genotoxic (Lave et al. 1982). Depending on the battery of tests they used, the lowest percent errors (false negatives plus false positives) was over 10%. Data were from the large international experiment reported by deSerres and Ashby (1981). One office of EPA has circulated a proposal (for use in establishing water quality standards) that would require two positive tests. This would increase the proportion of false negatives-- i.e., increase the consumer risk (U.S. Environmental Protection Agency 1982).

There is a theorem in statistical decision theory that states that the errors made using any decision rule are minimum for that set of data upon which the rule is based. This means that in testing an array of materials not included in the deSerres compilation, the overall error rate will be greater than the 10% reported by Lave et al. Drs. Weisberger and Williams have proposed a battery of tests for determining genotoxicity that was not tested in the deSerres operation, so we do not know its operating characteristics (Weisburger 1975; Weisberger, Williams 1981). Lave et al. suggest that false negatives and false positives not be given equal weight. They suggest that when testing new materials, to try to avoid the potential disasters that Peto spoke of, false negatives should be given more weight (because of their possible health consequences) than false positives. For a material already in use, there is some argument as to what differential weights should be given to false positives and false negatives. An ideal short term system would be one which yielded no false negatives, so that a material "passing" the battery could be given a clean bill of health. A material "failing" would go on (if commerically worthwhile) to a more sensitive (and probably more expensive) test or set of tests. However, since not all carcinogens are mutagens (or genotoxic) it is not likely that such a no-false-negatives battery can be developed.

MODEL IMPLICATIONS

The genotoxic-nongenotoxic division is meaningful
in how it impacts on establishing standards and in regulatory
behavior. Some scientists have seen a parallel between
the dichotomies of genotoxic-nongenotoxic and initiator-
promotor (Weisberger 1975; Williams 1982; Weisberger, Williams
1981). This is a simplification of the multistage theory
of carcinogenesis. The multistage theory envisions several
stages in the development of clinical disease. Richard
Peto, in writing about the mechanism of cigarette-smoke
carcinogenesis avoided this simplistic dichotomy and talked
about "early stage" and "late stage" carcinogens--asserting
his belief, based on the evidence from persons who quit
smoking, that cigarette smoke contains penultimate stage
carcinogens (Peto 1977). Day and Brown in their modeling
of the cancer process also indicate that several stages
are involved--and in looking at asbestos carcinogenesis
find that they are not able to clearly determine which
stages are affected by asbestos (Day, Brown 1980).

This difficulty about which stage or stages might be
affected is mirrored in the behavior of other materials as
carcinogens. If, as is sometimes argued, the dose-response
curve will be linear without a threshold at low doses only
for first stage carcinogens (loose translation: first
stage carcinogens are initiators, genotoxic materials)
then it becomes extremely difficult to explain the behavior
of 2-AAF--which seems to produce liver cancer (in rodents)
as if it were an early stage carcinogen (i.e., the dose-
response curve is linear and continues to increase after
treatment is stopped) and bladder cancers as if it were
a late stage carcinogen (i.e., a nonlinear dose response
curve which flattens out when treatments are stopped.) Or
DDT, which in most experiments appears to behave as a late
stage carcinogen (or promoter) and in one experiment by
Turasov seems to give a hyper-linear dose-response curve
in male mice, a curve form unexplained by any simple model
(Turasov et al. 1973).

Finally, we must consider that the concept of cancer
as a (somatic) genetic disease may need to be reexamined.
For example, what does one make of the result of Beatrice

Mintz in which transformed cells transplanted into mouse
embryos resulted not in cancer-bearing animals, but in
completely normal ones (Mintz 1976)? Is Emanuel Farber's
suggestion that at least one cell division is needed to
"fix" the genetic change, or transformation, an explanation
(Farber 1981)? What shall we make of Lijinsky's experiments
with a nitrosamine that at high doses produces cancers
at one site, and, at low doses at another--the whole cancer-
dose-response curve (as a time-related phenomenon) being
linear against dose (Lijinsky et al. 1981)?

     In a recent manuscript, Nicholas Day of IARC has put
forward several thoughts in relation to mathematical modeling
of the cancer process--particularly with respect to the use
of models in risk estimation (Day 1982). He reinforces
earlier work that led to our believing that "dose response
curves for late stage carcinogens may show different patterns
from dose-response curves for early carcinogens." He had
alluded to this in his earlier paper with Charles Brown
(Day, Brown 1980). There they show that the effect of
exposures to early stage carcinogens is acquired in a relatively short time and then does not diminish rapidly, even
after cessation of exposure. For example, for a first-
stage exposure at age 40, five years of exposure would,
by their calculations, produce 44% of the effect (excess
cancer risk over background) that a "remaining lifetime"
(40 years) of exposure would produce. On the other hand,
similar five-year exposure to a penultimate stage carcinogen
would give 11% of the excess cancer risk over background
compared to a remaining lifetime exposure. (See the 2-AAF
studies and liver cancers and bladder cancers as examples.)

     These results have serious implications for extrapola-
tion and for further experimentation; i.e., in attempts
to identify where in the carcinogenic process a material
fits and to identify materials other than complete carcinogens. I see the Brown-Day result as a possible unifying
force in helping sort out initiators, promoters, pro-car-
cinogens, proto-carcinogens, facilitators, etc. The Brown-
Day results lend support to the suggestion that the control
of late stage carcinogens can lead to relatively rapid
decline in cancer rates. Continuing exposures to late stage
carcinogens appear to be necessary until an irreversible
cancer process is triggered. Ending this exposure should
interrupt the process, so that, unless a preclinical transformation has already taken place, cancer will then not

develop. The experience with endometrial cancers and post-
menopausal estrogens is consistent with this formulation
of the cancer process. I find it important that Day and
Brown do not find it necessary to postulate the existence
of thresholds for "promoters" to explain this behavior
of late stage carcinogens although they do not preclude
this possibility (Day, Brown 1980).

The argument that late stage carcinogens may not require
the assumptions of a threshold to explain their behavior is
of considerable importance in standard setting. If, in fact,
Day and Brown are correct, then it seems to me that the distinction between genetic and nongenetic carcinogens becomes
far less important--at least for the purposes of disease
prevention. And disease prevention is why we want to do
risk assessment and standard setting. What the argument
says to me is that any distinction that might be meaningful
lies only between late stage carcinogens and uniquivocally
last stage carcinogens. Such an idea, however, offends
my concept of the continuity and uniformity of biological
systems. Day does not treat this issue--and, in fact,
remarks that in the present state of knowledge, perhaps
the best we can do, or the most we should attempt, is to
distinguish between early stage and late stage--rather
than consider a full multistage model.

PROBLEMS OF MODELS FOR DIETARY EFFECTS

Day is much concerned with risk as a function of time--
when he distinguishes between early stage and late stage
mechanisms. (Not materials! Recall that 2-AAF produces
liver tumors that indicate an early stage mechanism and
bladder tumors that indicate a late stage mechanism).
Differentiation between early stage and late stage, appears
to lie not in the material, but in the material-tissue
interaction, including perhaps modification of the material
by the liver, so that what gets to the bladder is something
other than what affects the liver. Day also cites examples
in which the carcinogenic action of two insults (materials,
physical processes, etc.) lead to a linear dose-response,
whereas exposure to one of the insults leads to a curvilinear
dose-response curve. Such a phenomenon is consistent with
a multistage process.

These observations raise serious questions about the

adequacy of existing models. How do we deal with multiple
exposures? There are examples of the multiplication of
effects--such as seen in the cigarette-smoking asbestos
worker. That phenomenon is consistent with the multistage
theory. But there are other combined exposures that don't
show a multiplicative effect. "Diet," of course, is a
shorthand for a very complex mixture of exposures. One
of the arguments for low-dose nonthreshold linearity lies
in the assumption that there are things already existing
in the environment (both initiators and promoters) that
have the same action or produce the same consequences as
the material of concern. The effect, then, of adding a
material of concern is merely to add some dose (of initiator,
or promoter) to an existing dose. For small additions
this leads to a linear response. The unresolved question
is how to equate doses. In a conceptual framework, however,
should we look upon the addition of new, suspect, materials
to the environment as adding to existing doses? Only when
some entirely different process must be called into play,
one that does not exist in nature (or is extremely rare,
perhaps) then the concept of additivity in dose may no
longer be germane to the modeling.

Because it appears that the action of diet in relation
to cancer is both as causal (in the sense of an agent like
fats being causal) and as preventive--i.e., the suggested
role for vitamin A (or its precursors) vitamin C, fiber,
etc. some modeling now needs to be developed for the anticancer action of "preventives." To my knowledge there
is very little work on the modeling of the behavior of
"preventers." Day remarks "The role of fiber in large
bowel cancer, Vitamin A and its precursors in lung cancer,
riboflavin and perhaps Vitamin A in esophagus and oral
cancer hold promise of providing more effective means of
prevention than identification of positive risk factors.
The form of the dose response, or dose protection, curves
for such agents can only be speculated on, but is likely
to demonstrate strong nonlinearity and the appearance of
threshold effect" (Day 1982). This implies that low doses
of "protectors" will provide little or no protection.
Perhaps some initial help in developing protection dose-
response models might be derived from looking at the effects
of dose of vitamins and of the trace elements in reducing
so-called deficiency diseases.

Considering other nutritionally related diseases (other

than some cancers) leads immediately to the consideration
of optimal levels of intake. A small amount of selenium
may be good. A large amount may lead to cancer (Griffin 1979;
Shamberger 1970; Shamberger, Frost 1969). In many situations
it may be important to try to uncover total health effects,
rather than the effects on a single disease, like, let
us say colon cancer (which may even be more than one disease).
Early full term pregnancy leads to reduced breast cancer.
Early sexual intercourse which leads to early full term
pregnancy also leads to increased cancer of the uterine
cervix. Higher fat intake (as Peto reported at this conference)
is correlated (internationally) with higher colo-rectal
cancer. Higher fat intake has been correlated with lower
total digestive system cancers (Segi et al. 1969; Segi
et al. 1977).

RESEARCH AND POLICY IMPLICATIONS

I will deal only a little with research and policy
implications. Peto made it clear that there are enormous
gaps in the knowledge we have about carcinogenic processes
associated with diet. Many anomalies and inconsistencies
need to be explained and understood. Perhaps the greater
understanding of these will lead to better model-building,
so that we might be able to do better risk assessments.
On a technical level in related areas, we need to develop
methods for putting together all the data, bacteria, mouse,
man-including the apparently contradictory studies. In
the epidemiology we need to take advantage of the confirma-
tion and better exposure estimates we can get by observing
special populations or population isolates. This means
studying not only Mormons (high meat and fat eaters) whose
breast cancer and colon cancer rates don't fit the pattern
one would expect from the international correlations, but
also studying Blacks in different areas in the United States.
One conference on cancer in Blacks has been held in the
United States, but it has not led me to much greater understanding of the high lung cancer and prostate cancer rates
in men and the still lower breast cancer incidence in black
women. If the "life-style" ideas are to be pursued "life-
style" will have to be better defined. When I think of
"life-style" as applied to me, I am able to count at least
seven different life-styles that I have lived. If I develop
some illness there should be no problem in finding a sufficiently "bad" life-style to blame it on. Interactions

between social class (which is largely determined by occupation, and which often determines occupation) and exposure to other life-style factors will have to be sorted out.

As for social policy implications, these are dealt with more fully in later papers in these proceedings, and I have only a few comments. First, if Peto's (and others) observation is correct that rapid and large reductions in cancer will occur if exposure to late stage carcinogens is substantially reduced (Peto 1977; Jick et al. 1979), then we need both research emphasis in finding late stage carcinogens, and social action so that the exposure to these materials will be very sharply reduced. Some of the recent arguments relating to genotoxic and nongenotoxic materials seem to lead to the reverse conclusion--i.e., that levels for late stage materials need not be so rigidly controlled as levels for other (early stage) carcinogens. That would be counterproductive.

In part, the actions that are taken within a society reflect basic social philosophy. A society largely concerned with human health will try to reduce what I have identified as "consumer risk." In the limited context here, this means settling upon testing techniques that minimize false negatives. Even in such a society, however, it must be recognized that some of the new products to be placed on the market may carry health benefits, so that a (false) positive label given to one of these materials will have a secondary deleterious health effect--i.e., health will not improve as rapidly as it might have had the material been put into use. There are obvious tertiary health benefits, too. Since richer is better than poorer, having a job is better than not having a job. Eating is better than not eating. This implies that the relative emphasis on preventive activities becomes a function of time and place, and other circumstances.

Social policy also derives from the philosophy of how responsibility is to be distributed among individuals, social organizations, corporate groups, government bodies, etc. The only comment I have concerning this is that the more complex and interdependent a society becomes, the more the societal institutions need to take on responsibilities. When I was growing up on a farm on Long Island, we drove a well-pipe into the ground down about 25-30 feet and we found safe, drinkable water. Industry has now spread out

of New York City to that part of Long Island and the ground-
water there is no longer drinkable. The water now used
is "city water"--from a central supply, filtered, aerated,
chlorinated, fluoridated, supplied by the community--at
a price. Thus the greater complexity of urban and sub-
urban living requires more government intervention. This
trend toward intervention has been going on for a long
time in the food area as each of us produces less of the
food we eat. If we wish to have people consume less fat,
we might achieve this goal by admonition (not a very good
way), by education (somewhat better--but still not as effective as we would perhaps like) or by government intervention
in modifying dairy price supports and in changing meat grad-
ing standards, or by graduated taxation on fat-containing
foods--the tax being graduated according to the fat content.
(This latter suggestion may not be as wild as it seems
on first hearing. This is now done with alcoholic beverages
and, in some cities and states, with cigarettes. Taxes
on these products are related to percent alcohol content,
and tar levels of the cigarettes.)

As a final issue within the social policy question,
one might ask how much scientific data need be at hand
to justify some action--ranging from official recommendations
to legislation or formal rules set out by the Federal Government. The amount and quality of data required seems to
vary with many factors, including one's personal social
philosophy. Scientists are rarely pleased or satisfied
with existing data. The recent NAS/NRC report on cancer
and diet is instructive along these lines because of its
apparent departure from the "don't do anything until you
are sure" approach. The report acknowledges the spotty
character and the weakness of the data concerning diet
and cancer and then goes on to support its recommendations
for dietary changes using an analogy to the cigarette smoke
issue. How much better off might we be today, the report
asks in effect, if we had taken action to reduce cigarette
smoking when the first data came to hand which showed the
strong cancer-smoking relationship. By analogy the report
urges dietary changes, although much of the data is still
weak or inconclusive. It seems to be arguing that for
very important problems, affecting large numbers of persons
that a policy that is low consumer risk oriented is the
most appropriate one to follow. The responses to the report
make it clear that this perception is not universally shared.

SUMMARY AND CONCLUSIONS

Improvements in health have taken place in the past--long before there was mathematical risk assessment. The implied promise of the new field of risk analysis is that the techniques will lead to even more rapid improvements in health. We shall have to wait to see if the promise is fulfilled or whether we will sometime in the future want to bring breach of promise suits against the risk assessors. The current models in cancer are thoughtful and seem to me to be derived from a sensible interpretation of existing human data. Improvements are needed to handle multiple exposures and "prevention-type" activity.

To estimate risks the mathematical modeling must bear a decent relationship to the biological processes--although it is quite clear that some good (but not perfect) estimation can be done without full knowledge of the intimate details of the biological processes. However, when implementing the knowledge of the biology to improve health social philosophy and social policy almost always intervene. The conclusion of whether the mouse or the bacterium is the more suitable model for man sometimes depends on social philosophy as much or more than it does on the science--especially if the science is new, or limited or not well understood. My personal social philosophy biases me toward being more concerned about consumer risk than producer risk, and to be more willing to move toward community or social action than some. I think this puts me close to the camp of the authors of the NAS report on diet and cancer. While I see community or corporate action as potentially far more effective, it is also not a complete substitute for individual action.

With respect to the newer biology involved in the short term tests, I like the ideas behind the short-term tests--but I believe regulatory recommendations based on distinctions being made between genotoxic and nongenotoxic carcinogens could lead to squandering a great deal of potential for disease prevention. If the nongenotoxic carcinogens make up the bulk of the promoters, and the control of promoters will lead to prompt health gains, it may be most reasonable to control the nongenotoxics more rigidly--not less rigidly. A strong health orientation leads me to want to see a testing battery developed that could produce a no-false-negatives situation--i.e., zero consumer risk--as the first stage in a fuller system for examining materials for their potential hazards--and worth. I don't anticipate that such a system will be soon developed.

By way of reply to the question in the title, I find that the mathematics, derived as it is from consideration of disease in both humans and animal systems, does give more meaning than mess. What arguments remain do not impress me as unresolvable, or fundamental.

Acknowledgement:

I am indebted to Peter LaGoy of Clement Associates for his considerable help in developing the bibliography for this paper.

References:

Armitage P, Doll R (1961). Stochastic models for carcinogensis. In Neyman J (ed): "Proceedings of the fourth Berkeley symposium on mathematical statistics and probability." Vol 4. Berkely and Los Angeles: University California Press, pp 19.

Armstrong BKl, Doll R (1975). Environmental factors and cancer incidence and mortality in different countries with special reference to dietary practices. Int J Cancer 15:617.

Ashby E (1979). "Reconciling Man with the Environment" Stanford, California: Stanford University Press, p 3.

Berg JW, Ross R, Labourette HB (1977). Economic status and survival of cancer patients. Cancer 39:467.

California Health and Welfare Agency (1982). "Carcinogen Identification Policy: A Statement of Science as a Basis of Policy" Sacramento, CA: California Department of Health Services.

Davis DL, Bridbord K, Schneiderman M (1981). Estimating cancer causes: Problems in methodology, production, and trends. In Peto R, Schneiderman M (eds): "Banbury Report 9: Quantification of Occupational Cancer": Cold Spring Harbor Laboratory pp 285.

Day NE (1982). Risk estimation models. Submitted for publication.

Day N.E. Brown C.C. (1980). Multistage models and primary prevention of cancer. J Natl Cancer Inst 64:977.

deSerres FJ, Ashby J (eds) (1981). "Evaluation of Short-term Tests for Carcinogens: Report of the International

Collaborative Program". Progress in Mutation Research:
Volume 1. New York: Elsevier/North Holland.

Doll R, Peto R (1981). The causes of cancer: Quantitative
estimates of avoidable risks of cancer in the United
States today. J Natl Cancer Inst 66:1191.

Farber E (1981). Chemical carcinogenesis. New Engl J
Med 305:1379.

Fox AJ, Adelstein AM (1978). Occupational mortality:
Work or way of life? J Epidemiol Community Health 32:73.

Gori GB (1980). The regulation of carcinogenic hazards.
Science 208:256.

Griffin AC (1979). Role of selenium in the chemoprevention of cancer. Adv Cancer Res 29:419.

Haenszel W (1961). Cancer mortality among the foreign-
born in the United States. J Natl Cancer Inst 26:37.

Haenszel W, Correa P (1975). Developments in the epidemiology
of stomach cancer over the past decade. Cancer Res 35:3452.

Handler P (1979). Dedication Address: Northwestern University
Cancer Center, Chicago, IL.

Higginson J (1980). Importance of environmental and occupational factors in cancer. J Tox Environ Health: 941.

Higginson J, and Muir CS (1979). Environmental carcinogenesis: Misconceptions and limitations to cancer control. J Natl Cancer Inst 63:1291.

Interagency Regulatory Liason Group (IRLG) (1979). Scientific bases for identification of potential carcinogens
and estimation of risks. J Natl Cancer Inst 63:244.

Jick H, Watkins RN, Hunter JR, Dinon BJ, Madsen S, Rothman
KJ, Walker AM (1979). Replacement estrogen and endometrial cancer. New Engl J Med 300:218.

Kegeles SS (1976). Relationship of sociocultural factors
to cancer. In Cullen JW, Fox BH, Isom RN (eds): "Cancer:
The Behavioral Dimensions" New York: Raven Press, pp 104.

Knowles JH (1977). The responsibility of the individual.
In Knowles JH (ed): "Doing Better and Feeling Worse:
Health in the United States," New York: W.W. Norton
and Co., Inc. pp 57.

Lambert CA, Netherton DR, Finison LJ, Hyde JN, Spaight
SJ (1982). Risk factors and lifestyle: A statewide
health-interview survey. N Engl J Med 306:1048.

Lave LB, Omenn GS, Heffernan KD, Dranoff G (1982). Analysis
of the cost-effectiveness of tier testing for potential
carcinogens. Presented at the First World Congress
on Toxicological and Environmental Health. Washington, D.C.
American College of Toxicology.

Lijinsky W, Reuber MD, Riggs CW (1981). Dose response

studies of carcinogenesis in rats by nitrosodiethyl-amine. Cancer Res 41:4997.

Mintz B (1976). Gene expression in neoplasia and differen-tiation. Harvey Lecture 71:193.

National Research Council (NRC). (1982). "Diet, Nutrition, and Cancer" Washington, D.C.: National Academy Press pp 204.

Nicholson WJ, Perkel G, Selikoff IJ, Seidman H (1981). Cancer from occupational asbestos expsoure: Projections 1980-2000. In Peto R, Schneiderman M (eds): "Banbury Report 9: Quantification of Occupational Cancer": Cold Spring Harbor Laboratory, pp 87.

Peto R (1977). Epidemiology, multistage models, and short-term mutagenicity tests. In Hiatt HH, Watson JD, Winsten JA (eds): "Origins of Human Cancer: Book C Human Risk Assessment." Cold Spring Harbor Conferences on Cell Proliferation Volume 4. Cold Spring Harbor Laboratory pp. 1403.

Peto R (1982). How will it be possible to progress from suggestions to reliable human evidence in nutrition. A paper presented at the Diet-Cancer workshop held at Cornell University, Ithaca, NY.

Segi M, Kurihera M, Matsuyama T (1969). "Cancer Mortality for Selected Sites in 24 Countries." No. 5 (1964-1965) Senadai: Tohaku University School of Medicine, Department of Public Health.

Segi M, Noye H, Segi R (1977). "The relation between food patterns and the death rates for stomach cancer and the cancer of the intestine and breast by countries" Japan: Segi Institute of Cancer Epidemiology.

Shamberger RJ (1970). Relationship of selenium to cancer. I. Inhibitory effect of selenium on carcinogenesis. J Natl Cancer Inst 44:931.

Shamberger RJ, Frost DV (1969). Possible protective effect of selenium against human cancer. Can Med Assoc J 100.

Shewhart WA (1931). "Economic Control of Quality of Manu-factured Product" New York: D. Van Nostrand Co., Inc. p 26.

Smith G, and Smyth JC, eds (1972). "The Biology of Affluence" Edinburgh: Oliver and Boyd

Squire R (1981). Ranking animal carcinogens: A proposed regulatory approach. Science 214:877.

Turasov V, Day NE, Tomatis L, Gati E, Charles RT (1973). Tumors in CF-1 mice exposed for six successive generations to DDT. J Natl Cancer Inst 51:983.

U.S. Department of Health and Human Services (USDHHS) (1982).

"The Health Consequences of Smoking": A report of the
    Surgeon General. Public Health Service, Office of Smoking
    and Health, Rockville, Maryland
U.S. Environmental Protection Agency (USEPA). (1982).
    "Additional USEPA Guidance for the Health Assessment
    of Suspect Carcinogens with Specific Reference to Water
    Quality Criteria" Draft Document for Comment
U.S. National Center for Health Statistics (USNCHS). (1982).
    Advance report of final mortality statistics, 1979.
    Monthly Vital Statistics Report 31, No. 6 Supplement
Weisburger JH (1975). Chemical carcinogenesis. In Casarett
    LJ, Doull J (eds): "Toxicology: The Basic Science
    of Poisons" New York: MacMillan Publishing Co., Inc.
    p 333.
Weisburger JH, Williams GM (1981). Carcinogen testing:
    Current problems and new approaches. Science 214:401.
Wildavsky A (1977). Doing better and feeling worse: The
    political pathology of health policy. In Knowles JH (ed):
    "Doing Better and Feeling Worse: Health in the United
    States," New York: W.W. Norton and Co., Inc. p 105.
William G (1982). Risk assessment and tumor promotion.
    This volume.
Wynder EL, Mabuchi K (1972). Etiological and preventive
    aspects of human cancer. Prev Med 1:300.
Ziegler RG, Blot WV, Hoover R, Blatner WA,
    Fraumeni JF Jr (1981). Protocol for a study of nutritional
    factors and the low risk of colon cancer in southern
    retirement areas. Cancer Res 41:3742.

PUBLIC POLICY

Diet, Nutrition, and Cancer:
From Basic Research to Policy Implications, pages 243–256
© *1983 Alan R. Liss, Inc., 150 Fifth Avenue, New York, NY 10011*

A DIET TO PREVENT COLON CANCER: HOW DO WE GET THERE FROM
HERE?

Gail McKeown-Eyssen, Ph.D.

Ludwig Institute for Cancer Research, Toronto
Branch and University of Toronto
Toronto, Ontario, Canada

Introduction

Evidence is accumulating that diet plays a role in the
etiology of a number of sites of human cancer (Grobstein
et al. 1982). Some scientists are beginning to modify their
own diets to reflect the scientific evidence. It is therefore reasonable to ask whether the time has arrived for a
public policy on diet. In deciding whether public policy is
now justified, the first consideration must be the quality
of the scientific evidence. Once this has been assured, the
best means of implementation, public education and/or modification of the food supply, can be determined and the optimal timing of the various actions can be ascertained.

This paper deals only with an evaluation of the scientific evidence for a dietary etiology of cancer. It takes
colon cancer as an example, because this is the major North
American site of cancer in both sexes in which diet has been
implicated, and considers the quality of the evidence for
two major hypotheses in colon cancer etiology, the role of
dietary fat and the role of dietary fibre.

In order to evaluate the quality of the current epidemiological evidence, the criteria proposed by Sackett (1976)
and Bradford-Hill (1967) have been applied. The first consideration is the nature of study designs (Sackett 1976).
The strength of the evidence from observational epidemiological research increases from descriptive studies, to case-
control comparisons, to cohort studies. Randomized human
experiments provide the most convincing evidence. The weight

of evidence from these study designs should be considered in the light of Bradford-Hill's principal criteria. Consistency of findings from different study designs and in different places and circumstances increases the certainty of the findings, as do the strength of any observed associations and the presence of dose-response relationships. Temporal relationships should be appropriate and findings should make both biological and epidemiological sense.

The Role of Fat

Dietary fat has received attention as a possible factor in the etiology of colon cancer. Descriptive studies have found a strong positive association between colon cancer mortality or incidence in different countries and the per capita availability in national diets of total fat (Armstrong and Doll 1975, Drasar and Irving 1973, Howell 1975, Knox 1977, Liu et al. 1979) and animal fat (Drasar and Irving 1973, Howell 1975), estimated from food balance sheets. In contrast, when fat consumption was assessed from food records and food analyses in Denmark and Finland, countries with a three-fold gradient in colon cancer incidence, no significant positive associations were found; indeed, total fat (International Agency for Research on Cancer 1977) and saturated fatty acids in the diet (Jensen et al. 1982) were negatively associated with colon cancer rates. Descriptive studies carried out within countries have also failed to find a positive association; total fat consumption assessed from food surveys was not associated with regional mortality within the UK (Bingham et al. 1979) or the USA (Enstrom 1975), or with colon cancer incidence of different ethnic groups in Hawaii (Kolonel et al. 1981).

Examination of the relationship between temporal trends in fat consumption and colon cancer mortality has also failed to provide support for the hypothesis that either total fat (Enig et al. 1978, Enstrom 1975) or animal fat (Enig et al. 1978, McMichael et al. 1979) is positively associated with colon cancer

Case-control studies have differed in the methods used to assess fat consumption and have provided mixed results. Only Jain and collegues (1980) have attempted to estimate levels of fat consumption by combining information from diet histories with information on the fat content of foods.

Total fat consumption estimated in this fashion was positively associated with colon cancer risk, and the group with
the highest fat consumption was at three times the risk of
colon cancer as the group with the least consumption
(relative risk=3.3). Philips (1975) found a significant
increase in risk associated with the eating of high saturated
fat foods when extreme categories of consumption were compared
(relative risk=2.7) but Dales et al. (1978), Modan et al.
(1975) and Higginson (1966) found no significant association.
The use of vegetable oil in cooking was negatively associated
with colon cancer in one investigation (Modan et al. 1975)
but not in three others (Haenszel et al. 1973, Higginson 1966,
Philips 1975) and no association was found for use of fried
foods (Graham et al. 1978, Higginson 1966, Philips 1975,
Wynder et al. 1969).

The biological plausibility of the role of fat in the
etiology of colon cancer is reflected in a number of theories
for the mechanism of action (Mastromarino 1981); these
include increased bile acid secretion into the gut, increased
metabolic activity of gut bacteria, increased secondary bile
acids in the colon, alteration of the immune system and
stimulation of the mixed-function oxidase system.

The Role of Fat-Containing Foods

Strong and consistent support for the hypothesis that
meat, especially beef, is positively associated with colon
cancer, comes from cross-sectional studies of international
colon cancer rates in relation to national diets (Armstrong
and Doll 1975, Howell 1975, Knox 1977, MacLennan et al. 1978,
Maruchi et al. 1977, Reddy et al. 1978). In contrast, no
differences in meat consumption were found between Denmark
and Finland, despite a three-fold gradient in their colon
cancer rates (Jensen et al. 1982), and no associations were
found in studies within countries of regional or ethnic
colon cancer rates in relation to meat (Kolonel et al. 1981,
Maruchi et al. 1977) or beef (Bingham et al. 1979, Blot
et al. 1976, Enstrom 1975) consumption. Within the USA,
Seventh Day Adventists who generally abstain from eating
meat have lower than average mortality from colon cancer
(Philips et al. 1980) but Mormons who do eat meat also have
low mortality (Lyon et al. 1980); within Britain, nuns who
do not eat meat had similar colon cancer rates to those who
did (Kinlen 1980). Studies of temporal trends have not

supported the hypothesis that meat (McMichael et al. 1979) or beef (Enstrom 1975) is positively associated with colon cancer mortality.

Case-control studies have provided equally conflicting results on the role of meat consumption. Philips (1975) detected a relative risk of 3.6 associated with the highest category of meat consumption twenty years previously, though not with current meat consumption, but five additional studies failed to find a significant association (Bjelke 1971, Dales et al. 1978, Graham et al. 1978, Haenszel et al. 1980, Higginson 1966). Indeed, a Japanese cohort study found that people who ate meat less than daily were at greater risk of colon cancer than those who ate meat more frequently (Hirayama 1981) and early results of a Norwegian cohort study indicated increased risk of colorectal cancer only among users of processed meats (Bjelke 1980).

The results of studies of beef consumption have also been inconsistent. Beef consumption was positively related to the risk of colon cancer in case-control studies of Hawaiian Japanese (highest reported relative risk=2.6) (Haenszel et al. 1973) and of Seventh Day Adventists (highest reported relative risk=3.1) (Philips 1975) but not in studies in Japan (Haenszel et al. 1980) or in the United States (Dales et al. 1978, Graham et al. 1978). The findings for other meats and for fish and poultry are equally variable.

Although dairy products are a source of fat, there is little consistent evidence of an association with colon cancer. National availability of milk and milk products estimated from food balance sheets was positively associated with international colon cancer rates (Armstrong and Doll 1975, Howell 1975) but these findings were not replicated when food consumption was surveyed in Denmark, Finland and New York (Jensen et al. 1982, MacLennan et al. 1978, Reddy et al. 1978). Within countries, studies of milk use in different regions of Japan (Maruchi et al. 1977) or among religious groups in California (Enstrom 1980) also failed to find positive associations with colon cancer. Indeed, Philips (1975) reported that cases of colon cancer used fewer milk products than controls and demonstrated a negative dose-response relationship with frequency of use (relative risk=0.3 for the maximum frequency of use). This finding contrasted with the results of a case-control study by

Wynder and colleagues (1969) who reported a positive association with milk use and with those of Wynder and Shigematsu
(1967) and Higginson (1966) who found no association.

International studies suggested a positive association
between colon cancer and availability of eggs (Armstrong and
Doll 1975, Drasar and Irving 1973, Howell 1975, Knox 1977,
Maruchi et al. 1977) but these findings were not confirmed
on comparison of food records from Denmark and Finland
(Jensen et al. 1982), in studies of regional colon cancer
within Japan (Maruchi et al. 1977) and within the USA
(Howell 1975), or in case-control studies (Wynder et al.
1969, Wynder and Shigematsu 1967).

The Role of Fibre

The hypothesis that a diet rich in fibre may protect
against colon cancer was proposed by Burkett and Trowell
(1975), who observed that Africans with a high fibre diet
experienced low death rates of bowel cancer. Although the
apparent protection conferred by cereals, vegetables and
fruit (see below) has been attributed, at least in part, to
their fibre content, few studies have attempted to estimate
fibre consumption. In one such study, a significant negative association was found between colon cancer incidence
in Denmark and Finland and both total dietary fibre,
(International Agency for Research on Cancer 1977, Jensen
et al. 1982) and individual types of fibre (International
Agency for Research on Cancer 1977); a strong negative association was reported between regional colon cancer mortality
within the UK and consumption of pentose, though not with
total dietary fibre (Bingham et al. 1979). In contrast,
national availability of crude fibre, cellulose and lignin,
was not correlated with international colon cancer incidence
(Drasar and Irving 1973). The relationship between temporal
trends in colon cancer mortality and levels of fibre consumption in the UK and the USA (McMichael et al. 1979) support the possibility of a protective effect.

One case-control study estimated crude fibre consumption in cases and controls (Jain et al. 1980) and found
significantly lower consumption in women with colon cancer
than in hospital, although not in neighbourhood, controls;
no significant differences were found for men. Dales et al.
(1978), Philips (1975) and Modan et al. (1975) identified

groups of high fibre foods but only Modan found a significant difference in their use between cases and controls.

Hypotheses of the biological action of fibre include increase in fecal bulk and dilution of carcinogens and promoters, modification of metabolic activity of gut bacteria and modification of the metabolism of carcinogens and/or promoters (Mastromarino 1981).

The Role of Fibre Containing Foods

Descriptive studies of international colon cancer patterns have consistently found negative associations between colon cancer rates and total cereal availability (Armstrong and Doll 1975, Howell 1975, Knox 1977, Maruchi et al. 1977), or cereal consumption (International Agency for Research on Cancer 1977, Jensen et al. 1982). Studies carried out within countries, however, have been less consistent; no association was found between cereal use and regional mortality in Japan (Maruchi et al. 1977), yet American Seventh Day Adventists have lower than expected death rates (Philips et al. 1980) and make extensive use of whole grains.

Case-control studies have not reported associations with total cereal use (Higginson 1966, Wynder and Shigematsu 1967), but cereals other than bread were negatively associated with colon cancer in Norway though not in the USA (Bjelke 1980). Rice was associated with an increased risk of colon cancer in two case-control studies (Haenszel et al. 1973 and 1980) but a cohort study in Japan reported consistent decreases in the risk of colon cancer with increased consumption of rice and wheat (Hirayama 1981).

National rates of colon cancer were not related to national levels of availability of fruit or of all vegetables (Armstrong and Doll 1975, Howell 1975, Knox 1977, Maruchi et al. 1977) but availability of legumes had a moderate negative association with national mortality in two investigations (Howell 1975, Knox 1977), though not in two others (Armstrong and Doll 1975, Maruchi et al. 1977). Further, no differences in fruit or vegetable consumption were found between Denmark and Finland, despite a three-fold gradient in cancer rates (Jensen et al. 1982). Within the United Kingdom, consumption of all vegetables and of green or yellow vegetables had a strong negative association with colon cancer mortality (Bingham et al. 1979) but no comparable associations were found with vegetables or fruit in Japan (Maruchi et al. 1977). Within the United States, Mormons and Seventh Day Adventists, religious groups with higher than average consumption of fruit and vegetables have low colon cancer rates (Enstrom 1980, Philips et al. 1980), but physicians from an Adventist medical school had similar mortality rates to physicians from a non-denominational school (Philips 1975), despite the presumed difference in their dietary habits. Temporal trends of fruit and vegetable consumption have not been associated with trends in colon cancer (McMichael et al. 1979).

Four case-control studies have confirmed the observation that consumption of one or more types of vegetable was negatively associated with colon cancer (Bjelke 1980, Graham et al. 1978, Haenszel et al. 1980, Modan et al. 1975) and Graham et al. (1978) reported a dose response relationship (minimum relative risk=0.6). In contrast, four other studies failed to find an association with vegetable use (Higginson 1966, Philips 1975, Wynder et al. 1969, Wynder and Shigematsu 1967) and Haenszel et al. (1973) found that, among Hawaiian Japanese, cases consumed more of certain vegetables than did controls. The relationship between vegetable consumption and risk of colon cancer assessed from prospective studies has also been inconsistent, as vegetable consumption was found to be associated with reduced risk of colorectal cancer in the USA but not in Norway (Bjelke 1980). Perhaps the most consistent finding has been the negative relationship seen in case-control studies between colon cancer and cruciferous vegetables, including cabbage (Graham et al. 1978, Modan et al. 1975), brussel sprouts and broccoli (Graham et al. 1978) and Japanese cabbage (Haenszel et al. 1980).

Evaluation of the Evidence

Although the strongest evidence would come from randomised trials designed to study the relationship between foods and colon cancer, none has yet been reported. Cohort studies have not supported the hypothesis, generated from descriptive epidemiology, that total meat consumption increases the risk of colon cancer (Hirayama 1981), although use of processed meats may increase risk (Bjelke 1980). Early findings from prospective studies of the role of vegetables in the USA and Norway have produced mixed results (Bjelke 1980). Case-

control studies have also provided inconsistent results on
the role of individual foods in the etiology of colon cancer,
and, where differences have been found between cases and
controls, relative risks have not been large.

Failure to find consistent, strong relationships does
not necessarily mediate against a dietary etiology of colon
cancer, however, because the findings may have arisen, at
least in part, from methodological limitations of the studies.
Several case-control studies have combined cases of colon
and rectal cancer, despite evidence that these conditions do
not have an identical etiology (Berg and Howell 1974). Some
may have underestimated relative risks by the inclusion among
hospital controls of patients with conditions, such as heart
disease or some cancers, which may have a dietary etiology.
All have attempted to ensure that temporal relationships
were appropriate by assessing diet before cancer was diagnosed but this has introduced difficulties in the dietary
measurement by the need to rely on subjects' recall of past
eating patterns. Finally, both cohort and case-control
studies may have been hampered by the possibility that diets
within communities have been too uniform to permit associations between diet and disease to be detected. Lack of variability in diet within countries may also account for the
failure of descriptive studies to confirm consistently some
strong associations between food and colon cancer which were
seen when international correlation studies exploited the
large variation in diet between nations.

Where Do We Go From Here?

Epidemiological studies suggest a role for diet in the
etiology of colon cancer. However, the evidence on the role
of specific foods is not conclusive, partly because of methodological limitations of the studies. Future research
should attempt to overcome these difficulties.

Randomized trials are needed to test the dietary hypotheses generated by observational epidemiology. Ultimately,
it may be desirable to conduct a dietary trial with cancer
incidence as the outcome; indeed, such a trial is planned to
evaluate the role of dietary supplementation by beta-carotene
in relation to total cancer incidence (Richard Peto, personal
communication). Trials of this nature require the study of
many thousands of persons over a number of years, so

researchers need endpoints other than cancer which might respond more quickly to dietary manipulation. Bruce et al. (1981) have planned studies of rates of occurence of adenomatous polyps, presumed precursors of colon cancer, in persons who have had previous adenomas removed during colonoscopy. After the initial polypectomy, patients are randomised into one of two dietary groups and followed for a period of two years to ascertain the occurence of new adenomatous lesions. Two types of dietary intervention are planned; in the first, subjects will be asked to eat each day a high fibre snack containing 25 grams of bran fibre or a placebo snack containing about 5 grams of fibre; the second intervention will attempt to reduce the fat content of the diet to about 15% of total calories in the intervention group, while leaving the control subjects on a diet conforming to Canada's Food Guide, with approximately 40% of calories taken as fat. Other endpoints are also possible; Decosse (personal communication) has examined both regression of rectal polyps and cell kinetics in patients with familial polyposis after dietary supplementation with vitamin C. The presence of micronuclei in the cells of colon crypts, a marker genetic damage (Heddle et al. 1982), may also serve as an outcome in randomised trials of dietary manipulation in animals and man.

Case-control studies could also be based on cases with early markers in the disease process (colon polyps, nuclear abnormalities, or cell kinetics). In such studies, the limitations of some previous case-control studies should be avoided by ensuring that controls are free of potentially diet related conditions and that attempts are made to obtain accurate assessments of diet. We are currently conducting such a study in a Toronto clinic where sigmoidoscopy is used to screen asymptomatic subjects for colon polyps. Prior to the sigmoidoscopic examination, all subjects participate in a dietary enquiry, supplemented by laboratory measures designed to reflect food intake. Urinary excretion of 3-methylhistidine is used as a marker for consumption of muscle protein (Jacobson et al. 1982) and fecal fat and fibre may also be used to reflect dietary intakes. The diets of subjects found to have adenomatous polyps will be compared with those of controls found to be free of intestinal lesions and of other potentially diet related conditions.

Until results of future research are available, public policy on diet must be based on a synthesis of current

knowledge of the relationship between diet and cancer. Such
dietary recommendations have recently been published by an
expert committee of the National Academy of Sciences
(Grobstein et al. 1982). Their guidelines proposed that the
consumption of fats be reduced in the average American diet,
stressed the importance of including fruits, vegetables and
whole grain cereal products in the daily diet, recommended
minimal consumption of foods preserved by salt curing or
smoking, proposed that efforts continue to minimize contamination of foods with carcinogens from any source, encouraged
efforts to identify mutagens in food, and proposed that, if
alcoholic beverages are consumed, it be done in moderation.
These recommendations agree with those published by the
National Cancer Centre Research Institute in Japan (Sugimura
1982) and by the Department of National Health and Welfare
in Canada (Murray and Rae 1979). The similarity between the
American and Canadian recommendations is of interest as the
latter were based on the relationship between diet and heart
disease, rather than diet and cancer.

Because of the present lack of conclusive evidence on
the relationship between diet and cancer, it is essential
for the credibility of the scientific community that advice
given to the public at this time should be seen as preliminary. This approach was taken by the National Academy of
Sciences who referred to their recommendations as interim
guidelines. They stressed that "the weight of evidence
suggests that what we eat during our lifetime strongly influences the probability of developing certain kinds of
cancer but that it is not now possible, and may never be
possible, to specify a diet that protects all people against
all forms of cancer." The committee also explained that
future research is likely to provide new insights into the
relationship between diet and cancer and therefore suggested
that the National Cancer Institute establish mechanisims for
review of the dietary guidelines at least every five years.
When the preliminary nature of present recommendations is
clearly understood, members of the public, government and
industry will be in a position to weigh appropriately the
personal and economic implications. Nevertheless, dietary
recommendations based on the current leads from scientific
research are desirable, despite their necessarily tentative
nature, because they form the basis of a nutritionally sound
diet which has the potential of reducing cancer rates in
North America.

Armstrong B, Doll R (1975). Environmental factors and cancer incidence and mortality in different countries, with special reference to dietary practices. Br J Cancer 15:617.

Berg JW, Howell MA (1974). The geographic pathology of bowel cancer. Cancer 34:807.

Bingham S, Williams DRR, Cole TJ, James WPT (1979). Dietary fibre and regional large-bowel cancer mortality in Britain. Br J Cancer 40:456.

Bjelke E (1971). Case-control study of cancer of the stomach, colon, and rectum. In Clark RL, Cumley RC, McCay JE, Copeland MM (eds): "Oncology 1970. Volume 5: A. Environmental Causes. B. Epidemiology and Demography. C. Cancer Education," Chicago: Yearbook Medical Publishers, p 320.

Bjelke E (1980). Epidemiology of colorectal cancer, with emphasis on diet. In Davis W, Harrap KR, Stathopolous G (eds): "Human cancer. Its charactarization and treatment. International Congress Series 484," Amsterdam: Excerpta Medica, p 158.

Blot WJ, Fraumeni JF, Stone BJ, McKay F (1976). Geographic patterns of large bowel cancer in the United States. J Natl Cancer Inst 57:1225.

Bradford-Hill A (1967). "Principles of Medical Statistics." London: The Lancet Limited, p 302.

Bruce WR, McKeown-Eyssen G, Ciampe A, Dion PW, Boyd N (1981). Strategies for dietary intervention studies in colon cancer. Cancer 47:1121.

Burkitt DP, Trowell HC (1975). "Refined carbohydrate foods and disease. Some implications of dietary fibre." London, New York and San Francisco: Academic Press, p 356.

Dales LG, Friedman GD, Ury HK, Grossman S, Williams SR (1978). A case-control study of relationships of diet and other traits to colorectal cancer in American Blacks. Am J Epidemiol 109:132.

Drasar BS, Irving D (1973). Environmental factors and cancer of the colon and breast. Br J Cancer 27:167.

Enig MG, Munn RJ, Keeney M (1978). Dietary fat and cancer trends - a critique. Fed Proc 37:2215.

Enstrom JE (1975). Colorectal cancer and consumption of beef and fat. Br J Cancer 32:432.

Enstrom JE (1980). Health and dietary practices and cancer mortality among California Mormons. In Cairns J, Lyon JL, Skolnick M (eds): "Cancer Incidence in Defined Populations. Banbury Report 4," Cold Spring Harbor Laboratory, p 69.

Graham S, Dayal H, Swanson M, Mittelman A, Wilkinson G (1978). Diet in the epidemiology of cancer of the colon and rectum. J Natl Cancer Inst 61:709.

Grobstein C, Cairns J, Berliner R, Broitman SA, Campbell TC, Gussow JD, Kolonel LN, Kritchevsky D, Mertz W, Miller AB, Prival MJ, Slaga T, Wattenberg L, Sugimura T (1982). "Diet, Nutrition, and Cancer." Washington: National Academy Press.

Haenszel W, Berg JW, Segi M, Kurihara M, Locke FB (1973). Large-bowel cancer in Hawaiian Japanese. J Natl Cancer Inst 51:1765.

Haenszel W, Locke FB, Segi M (1980). A case-control study of large bowel cancer in Japan. J Natl Cancer Inst 64:17.

Heddle JA, Blakey DH, Duncan AMV, Goldberg MT, Newmark H, Wargovich MJ, Bruce WR (1982). Micronuclei and related nuclear abnormalities as a short-term assay for colon carcinogens. Ban Rep 13. In press.

Higginson J (1966). Etiological factors in gastrointestinal cancer in man. J Natl Cancer Inst 37:527.

Hirayama T (1981). A large-scale cohort study on the relationship between diet and selected cancers of digestive organs. In Bruce WR, Correa P, Lipkin M, Tannenbaum SR, Wilkins TD (eds): "Gastrointestinal Cancer: Endogenous Factors. Banbury Report 7," Cold Spring Harbor Laboratory, p 409.

Howell MA (1975). Diet as an etiological factor in the development of cancers of the colon and rectum. J Chronic Dis 28:67.

International Agency for Research on Cancer Intestinal Microecology Group (1977). Dietary fibre, transit-time, faecal bacteria, steroids, and colon cancer in two Scandinavian populations. Lancet:207.

Jacobson EA, Newmark HL, McKeown-Eyssen G, Bruce WR (1982). Urinary 3-methylhistidine excretion as an estimate of meat consumption. Submitted to Am J Clin Nut.

Jain M, Cook GM, David FG, Grace MG, Howe GR, Miller AB (1980). A case-control study of diet and colo-rectal cancer. Int J Cancer 26:757.

Jensen OM, MacLennan R, Wahrendorf J (1982). Diet, bowel function, faecal characteristics and large bowel cancer in Denmark and Finland. Nutr Cancer. In press.

Kinlen LJ (1980). Mortality in relation to abstinence from meat in certain orders of religious sisters in Britain. In Cairns J, Lyon JL, Skolnick M (eds): "Cancer incidence in defined populations, Banbury Report 4," Cold Spring Harbor Laboratory, p 135.

Knox EG (1977). Foods and diseases. Br J Prev Soc Med 31:71.

Kolonel LN, Hankin JH, Lee J, Chu SY, Nomura AMY, Ward Hinds M (1981). Nutrient intakes in relation to cancer incidence in Hawaii. Br J Cancer 44:332.

Liu K, Moss D, Persky V, Stamler J, Garside D, Soltero I (1979). Dietary cholesterol, fat, and fibre, and colon-cancer mortality. Lancet:782.

Lyon JL, Gardner JW, West DW (1980). Cancer risk and life-style: cancer among Mormons from 1967 to 1975. In Cairns J, Lyon JL, Skolnick M (eds): "Cancer incidence in defined populations, Banbury Report 4," Cold Spring Harbor Laboratory, p 3.

MacLennan R, Jensen OM, Mosbech J, Vuori H (1978). Diet, transit time, stool weight, and colon cancer in two Scandinavian populations. Am J Clin Nutr 31:S239.

Maruchi N, Aoki S, Tsuda K, Tanaka Y, Toyokawa H (1977). Relation of food consumption to cancer mortality in Japan, with special reference to international figures. Gann 68:1.

Mastromarino AJ (1981). Summary of research progress. Cancer Bull 33:156.

McMichael AJ, Potter JD, Hetzel BS (1979). Time trends in colo-rectal cancer mortality in relation to food and alcohol consumption: United States, United Kingdom, Australia and New Zealand. Int J Epidemiol 8:295.

Modan B, Barell V, Lubin F, Modan M, Greenberg RA, Graham S (1975). Low-fiber intake as an etiologic factor in cancer of the colon. J Natl Cancer Inst 55:15.

Murray TK and Rae J (1979). Nutrition recommendations for Canadians. Can Med Assoc J 120:1241.

Philips RL (1975). Role of life-style and dietary habits in risk of cancer among Seventh-Day Adventists. Cancer Res 35:3513.

Philips RL, Kuzma JW, Lotz TW (1980). Cancer mortality among comparable members versus nonmembers of the Seventh-Day Adventist Church. In Cairns J, Lyon JL, Skolnick M (eds): "Cancer Incidence in Defined Populations. Banbury Report 4," Cold Spring Harbor Laboratory, p 93.

Reddy BS, Hedges A, Laakso K, Wynder EL (1978). Fecal constituents of a high-risk North American and a low-risk Finnish population for the development of large bowel cancer. Cancer Lett 4:217.

Sackett DI (1976). The diagnosis of causation. Mead Johnson Symposium on Perinatal and Developmental Medicine No 9. Vale, Colorado, p 3.

Sugimura T (1982). Tumor initiators and promoters associated with ordinary foods. In Arnott MS, van Eys J, Wang YM (eds): "Molecular Interrelations of Nutrition and Cancer," New York: Raven Press, p 3.

Wynder EL, Kajitani T, Ishikawa S, Dodo H, Takano A (1969). Environmental factors of cancer of the colon and rectum. Cancer 23:1210.

Wynder EL, Shigematsu T (1967). Environmental factors of cancer of the colon and rectum. Cancer 20:1520.

Diet, Nutrition, and Cancer:
From Basic Research to Policy Implications, pages 257–268
© *1983 Alan R. Liss, Inc., 150 Fifth Avenue, New York, NY 10011*

RDA's - ROLE IN PREVENTION

M.C. Cheney, Ph.D.
P.J. Steele, M.Sc.
Health Protection Branch
Department of National Health and Welfare
Ottawa, Canada. K1A 0L2

Officially accepted statements of the needs of populations for essential nutrients are a fundamental requirement for governments interested in the nutritional well-being of their people. Thus the first recommended dietary allowances (RDA) in the United States were developed in 1941 at a time when the government was concerned about the adequate nourishment of its civilian population and armed forces (Roberts, 1958). Since the RDA were first published by the National Academy of Sciences (Food and Nutrition Board, 1943) they have been continually revised by a series of committees.

Recommended nutrient intakes were originally developed to be used as guides for the planning and procuring of food supplies for population groups (Harper, 1979). The original focus of the recommendations was, and still is, the prevention of nutrient deficiencies by meeting the nutritional requirements of a population. But the definition of nutrient requirement has shifted over the years from an amount of a nutrient required to prevent deficiency to the current definition in the 1982 Recommended Nutrient Intakes for Canadians - "the amount of a nutrient that meets an individual's need, described as the establishment and maintenance of a reasonable level of the nutrient in body tissues or stores" (Canada. NHW, in press).

The 1980 edition defines the RDA as follows: "Recommended Dietary Allowances (RDA) are the levels of intake of essential nutrients considered, in the judgement of the Committee on Dietary Allowances of the Food and Nutrition Board on the basis of available scientific evidence, to be adequate to meet the known nutritional needs of practically all healthy persons" (Food and Nutrition Board, 1980).

Recommended nutrient intakes are intended to apply to healthy populations. They do not cover situations in which nutrient needs are altered due to, for example, disease, disorder or medication and which require individual attention. They do not deal with the role of long term nutrient intake in the pathogenesis of chronic diseases such as atherosclerosis and cancer. In 1980, the Committee on Dietary Allowances, in examining this issue concluded that the evidence linking nutrient intakes with chronic diseases was not of a nature to permit the basing of recommendations on disease prevention. Three years later, the Committee for the Revision of the Dietary Standard for Canada came to a similar conclusion.

In considering the role of the RDA in attempting to reduce the incidence of cancer, the currently available evidence linking nutrients to cancer will be compared with the evidence used to establish the RDA. This may explain why the RDA are not based on disease prevention. Possible conflicts between the current objectives of the RDA and cancer prevention will be explored and the impact on public policy if the goal of cancer prevention results in major changes in the RDA will be discussed.

Human Nutrient Requirements: Kinds of Evidence

Estimates of nutrient requirements are based on three kinds of evidence - epidemiological studies, controlled human studies and animal experimentation (Table 1) (Food and Nutrition Board, 1980; Sandstead, 1981).

Epidemiological data play a role in determining requirements. Early estimates of human nutrient needs were frequently based on observed intakes of apparently healthy subjects. One pitfall of this approach was pointed out by Hindhede (1913) in criticizing Voit's recommendations for protein intake based on the diet of German brewery workers. These men were found to die at an earlier age than the general population. Now, they probably would be considered the victims of over-consumption since it was established that they consumed on average 190 g protein, 73 g fat and 600 g carbohydrate daily for a total of over 3700 calories.

Table 1: Comparison of Types of Data Used For Estimating Dietary Requirements and for Relationship of Nutritional Factors to Cancer

Dietary Requirements	Nutrition and Cancer
Epidemiological Data	Epidemiological Data
. nutrient intake of healthy people	. descriptive
. nutritional status	. aggregate correlation data
. intervention	. case-control studies
	. cohort studies
	. intervention
Controlled Human Studies	
. balance techniques	
. depletion-repletion	
. metabolic function	
Animal Experimentation	Animal Experimentation
. nutrient deficiency in relation to growth, biochemical and physiological parameters	. short term studies
	. long term bioassay

Intervention to correct nutrient deficiencies has provided useful estimates of dietary levels of nutrients above which deficiencies are unlikely and data on nutrient intakes of free-living populations are used to evaluate recommended intakes based on experimental data. Epidemiological studies are, however, considered to be an insensitive method of determining nutrient requirements because dietary intakes cannot be measured accurately and therefore do not correlate well with laboratory and clinical measures of nutritional status.

Although controlled human studies are inevitably short term and limited in the number of subjects, their results can be extremely useful, especially when used in conjunction with the evidence from epidemiological studies and animal experimentation. In these studies the actual intakes of nutrients are known and definite endpoints or indicators of nutritional status are measured e.g. the quantity of a nutrient required to achieve equilibrium, to cure symptoms of deficiency, to restore or normalize metabolic function, to produce certain tissue levels, to permit stores to accumulate, etc. Animal experiments provide useful data on the quantitative effects of different physiological conditions and on the effects of nutrient interactions on requirements.

Nutrients Linked to Cancer: Kinds of Evidence

There are two principal kinds of evidence linking nutrients with the incidence of cancer - laboratory studies, and epidemiological studies (Table 1) (Committee on Diet, Nutrition and Cancer, 1982), p. 3-9. The results of these studies have not to date provided the type of data needed to make quantitative recommendations regarding nutrient intakes. This is not surprising considering the obscurity of the relationships between diet and degenerative and malignant diseases. Since cancer may be associated with dietary patterns that extend over a number of years and probably involve both nutrients and non-nutrients, it is not possible to carry out controlled human studies of the type which has provided much of the recent information about nutrient requirements.

The type of epidemiological studies which have shown an association between diets and/or nutrients and cancer include a) descriptive studies of disease patterns and dietary intakes b) aggregate correlation data between exposure and outcome, c) case-control studies comparing the diet of cancer patients with that of non-cancerous controls, d) cohort studies of cancer occurrence rates in two groups of individuals with different dietary histories and e) intervention studies (although these are rare).

Of these, the first two types of studies are merely suggestive and do not reflect true individual associations between nutrient intake and cancer. Cohort and intervention studies are very useful but few exist. Hence, in drawing conclusions about nutrient-cancer relationships particular attention is placed on the results of case-controlled studies. These have a number of weaknesses, an important one being the difficulty in obtaining accurate nutrient intake data.

In studying patients with cancer, the past diet may be more relevant than the present. However, it is extremely difficult to determine past dietary intakes. Even when previous dietary records exist for patients, they cannot be assumed to reflect the usual diet during the intervening years. In a recent study of consumers, 40% claimed to have made changes in their eating habits in the past year (Canada. NHW, 1979). Group dietary data such as national per capita consumption or disappearance, and household food inventories do provide retrospective information for a population but they do not account for differences in individual distribution and cannot be used in studies of individuals.

None of the methods of determining individual dietary intakes is perfect. All depend on the skill of the interviewer and the co-operativeness and alertness of the subject. Recent recall such as the 24 hour recall is of too short duration to give an estimate of the usual intake of the individual (Anon, 1976). Seven day and four day records can be used in small surveys but the requirement to record all foods eaten may modify dietary patterns for ease of recording. A diet history is limited to the intakes of certain foods and may result in important omissions (Young et al., 1952). Associations with vitamins A and C are often derived from frequency of fresh fruit and vegetable consumption. Not only is this likely to underestimate the quantities of vitamins consumed but it ignores the point that foods contain many substances in addition to micronutrients. It is probable that levels of vitamins are strongly correlated positively or negatively with those of other factors. Thus, vitamin C intakes reflect intakes of substances in fruit and vegetables; vitamin A, the intake of vegetables.

The calculation of nutrient intakes from dietary data is fraught with inaccuracies. Faulty estimates of the amounts of foods eaten are the first source of error. The second is in the use of tables of food composition to estimate the quantities of nutrients. These tables list average values which may not be representative of the foods eaten (Watt, 1980). For example, evidence is accumulating which suggests that the vitamin C values for vegetables in USDA Handbook No. 8 are not applicable to vegetables available in Canada (Pelletier et al., 1977; University of Guelph, unpublished data).

Potential Conflicts in Objectives

Should the evidence ever be considered sufficient to permit the development of recommended nutrient intakes based on reduction in cancer risk, this could conceivably result in increases in the recommended nutrient intakes for certain nutrients and upper limits on the intakes of other nutrients. The concept of safe ranges of nutrient intake has been considered by both the American and Canadian committees but the data establishinq the upper range of safe intakes are limited or lacking for most nutrients and where available, are based on toxicity rather than reduction in risk of disease (Canada, NHW, in press; Food and Nutrition Board, 1980). The safe range of intake in terms of multiples of the recommended intake varies from nutrient to nutrient and may be much narrower in the case of the macro-nutrients.

In the National Academy of Sciences report, Diet, Nutrition and Cancer (1982, p. 1-5), it was stated that evidence from both epidemiological and laboratory studies suggests that high intakes of protein may be associated with an increased risk of cancers of certain sites, although due to the dearth of available data, firm conclusions were not drawn.

In the hypothetical situation that it is eventually demonstrated that a lower protein intake is protective and that it would be prudent to recommend an upper limit on protein intakes, the impact of such a recommendation on vunerable groups within a population would have to be carefully examined. RDA are used in planning food supplies and food assistance programs. Incorporating an upper limit in the RDA for protein might increase the risk that the needs of all in a group will not be met especially if the limit was expressed as a proportion of energy. Of particular concern would be women of child-bearing age, elderly women, and those who are intermittently or chronically restricting their energy intake to lose weight. Recent surveys in the United States (USDA, 1980; USDHEW, 1977) and Canada (Canada. NHW, 1973) indicate that the average protein intake of young and elderly women exceed the recommended intake by only a small margin, and are below the levels that might be cause for concern about excessive intakes.

RDA are also be used to develop nutrition education programs; an upper limit on protein would raise the possibility of a recommendation to the public for moderate protein restriction. The risk that such a recommendation could be interpreted and applied inappropriately by individuals and that significant protein malnutrition could result must be considered. Recent evidence of delayed growth and puberty onset in a group of adolescents whose parents were following prudent diets (Pugliese et al., 1982) indicates the extremes to which public recommendations may be taken.

Establishment of upper limits could be in conflict with the basic objective of the RDA which is to meet the known nutritional needs of practically all healthy persons. The RDA seem extremely generous when compared to the actual experiences of the developing world where children grow more slowly than in North America but do not seem less healthy (Walker and Walker, 1981). While there is some question whether any benefit is derived from such generous allowances, would North Americans be prepared to accept anything less than maximal growth in their children?

Impact on Public Policy

The uses of recommended nutrient intakes have expanded well beyond their original intended use of planning and procuring food supplies for population groups (Table 2). Because of this, they could be a potent tool for the implementation of dietary change. Consider the impact of the RDA in the United States. In line with their original purpose, they are used as a basis for menus in hospitals and other institutions and in planning diets for the military. RDA are used as guides in the evaluation of data on nutrient intakes obtained from dietary surveys such as the Nationwide Food Consumption Survey. Federally funded feeding programs such as the National School Lunch Program have guidelines that meals served to program participants provide a certain proportion of the RDA. The RDA are used as guides in the preparation of nutrition education materials. Changes in the RDA would affect institutional diets, evaluation of survey results, criteria for feeding programs and nutrition education programs.

A set of RDA termed the U.S. RDA have been developed for regulatory purposes and are used as standards for the nutrition labelling of foods and in the Food Fortification Policy (United States, 1980). The U.S. RDA are used to establish significant levels of nutrient loss for the purposes of restoration, to define nutritional inferiority in a replacement for a traditional food and to set levels of nutrients relative to energy to be present in the food to balance the vitamin, mineral and protein content. Adjustments in the RDA if reflected in the U.S. RDA could have a marked impact on the composition of foods and the information on food labels.

Table 2: Uses of Recommended Nutrient Intakes

. Planning and Procuring Food Supplies
. Evaluating Nutritional Adequacy of Food Supplies
. Evaluating Dietary Survey Information
. Establishing Standards for Food Assistance Programs
. Developing Nutrition Education Programs
. Developing Nutritional Quality Criteria For Foods
. Establishing Criteria for Nutrition Labelling

Recommended nutrient intakes are used as guides in evaluating the adequacy of the food supply to meet the nutritional needs of the population and thus may affect national agricultural and food policies. For example, in Canada, the recommended intake of vitamin C will be increased in the 1982 revision of the standard to 60 mg for the adult male and 45 mg for the adult female. This may not seem significant in the United States where the RDA for vitamin C has been as high as 75 mg. When the Committee on Dietary Allowances set the RDA for vitamin C at 60 mg in 1980, they stated that this intake would not be difficult to achieve from the available food supply. However, the Canadian situation may be somewhat different.

A comparison of the recommend intakes of vitamin C and food supply availability is given in Table 3. The estimated per capita recommended intake of vitamin C adjusted for age and sex of the Canadian population, and incorporating a 25% increase for smokers is 56 mg. The food supply provides 115 mg vitamin C per capita but when this is reduced by estimates for losses to the household level and for cooking of vegetables, the amount of vitamin C available on a per capita basis is only 20% above the per capita recommended intake. When the mean intake of a population is equal to the recommended intake, 50% of the population could consume less than the recommended intake. This does not mean that 50% of the population will be deficient but if the current food supply contains insufficient quantities of vitamin C to supply the recommended nutrient intake this obviously has implications for government policies.

Table 3:   A Comparison of a Weighted Recommended Intake of
            Vitamin C, with the Estimated Available Supply of
            Vitamin C in Canada

Recommended Intake for Population	Vitamin C (mg/d)
Composite RNI (Vitamin C) [1]	48
Add. Requirement for Smokers [2]	+8
Total per capita	56
Estimated Available Supply	
Per Capita Disappearance (Vitamin C) [3]	115
Estimated retail and household losses [4]	-35
Estimated cooking losses [5]	-14
Total per capita	66

[1] Recommended intake of Vitamin C based on recommendations for age and sex categories as set out in the Recommended Nutrient Intakes of Canadians (Canada, NHW, in press) and adjusted for the population distribution by age and sex in 1979 (Canada. Stats. Can., 1981)

[2] Additional vitamin C requirements for smokers (Canada. NHW, in press) corrected for the proportion of smokers in the adult population (Canada. NHW., 1981).

[3] Calculation of mean vitamin C disappearance based on 5 year (1975-79) apparent per capita food consumption Canada. Ag. Can., 1981).

[4] Total estimates include 20% estimated loss at the wholesale and retail levels based on percentage differences between vitamin C disappearance and vitamin C availability from the Family Food Expenditure survey (Canada. Ag. Can., 1981)

[5] Estimates based on cooking losses of 30% for potatoes (Pelletier et al., 1977) and 35% for other vegetables that are usually cooked (Bender, 1978).

Dietary Recommendations
_____

Although the data linking nutrient intakes with risk of cancer are qualitative at the present time, this does not rule out action at the official level to reduce risks. The situation is rather analogous to that of the relationship between, diet, nutrient intake and cardiovascular disease which has been under study for decades. Evidence points to the advisability of dietary modifications for persons at risk for coronary heart disease and other conditions related to elevated blood lipids. The Committee on Dietary Allowances (Food and Nutrition Board, 1980) accordingly recommended that in the high risk population, total fat intake should not exceed 35% of energy intake and about 8-10% of energy should be from polyunsaturated (essential) fatty acids. The Committee were not prepared to make a blanket recommendation for dietary change for the whole population. They did, however, give guidelines similar to the above, "for individual consideration" - total fat intake reduced to not more than 35% of energy and an upper limit on polyunsaturates of 10% of energy.

In contrast, the Canadian Committee revising the recommended nutrient intakes decided that there was insufficient evidence upon which to base a quantitative recommendation or even guideline for maximum fat intake. But, official nutrition recommendations independant of the Recommended Nutrient Intakes for Canadians call for a reduction in the consumption of fat to 35% of energy, to include a source of linoleic acid in the diet, and consumption of a diet which emphasizes whole grain cereals, fruits and vegetables and minimizes alcohol, salt and refined sugars (Canada. NHW, 1978).

The Scandinavians first adopted dietary recommendations in 1968. Now Sweden has combined a statement of recommended nutrient intakes with recommendations for dietary patterns into one publication, Swedish Nutrition Recommendations (1981). The aim of these recommendations is to define the basis for planning a diet that satisfies the primary nutritional requirements, i.e. the RDA, that provide the prerequisites for general good health and that reduce the risk of disease caused by faulty diets.

The authors thank C.A. Scythes M.Sc., for her valuable assistance in preparing the manuscript.

Anon (1976). The validity of 24-hour dietary recalls. Nutr. Rev 34 (10):310.

Bender AE (1978). "Food Processing and Nutrition", New York: Academic Press p 43, 99.

Canada. Agriculture Canada (1981). "The Apparent Nutritive Value of Food Available for Consumption in Canada 1960-75", Ottawa: Information Services, p 46.

Canada. Department of National Health and Welfare (in press). "Recommended Nutrient Intakes for Canadians", Ottawa: Minister of Supply & Services.

Canada. Department of National Health and Welfare (1981). "The Health of Canadians. Report of the Canada Health Survey", Ottawa: Minister of Supply and Services.

Canada. Department of National Health and Welfare (1979). "Report of Nutrition Concepts and Evaluation Study", Ottawa: Minister of Supply and Services.

Canada. Department of National Health and Welfare (1978). Nutrition Recommendations for Canadians. Ottawa: Health Services and Promotion Branch, Nutrition Education Unit.

Canada. Department of National Health and Welfare (1973). "Nutrition Canada National Survey", Ottawa: Information Canada.

Canada. Statistics Canada (1981). "Apparent Per Capita Food Consumption in Canada Part II 1979", Ottawa: Minister of Supply and Services.

Committee on Diet, Nutrition and Cancer (1982). "Diet, Nutrition and Cancer", Washington: National Academy Press.

Food and Nutrition Board (1943). Recommended dietary allowances. National Research Council report and circulation series no. 115.

Food and Nutrition Board (1980). "Recommended Dietary Allowances", 9th edition, Washington: National Research Council, National Academy of Sciences.

Harper AE (1979). Uses and misuses of recommended dietary allowances. N Y State J Med 79(5):806.

Hindhede M (1913). "Protein and Nutrition: An investigation", London: Ewart, Seymour and Company, p 15.

Pelletier O, Nantel C, Leduc R, Tremblay L, Brassard R (1977). Vitamin C in potatoes prepared in various ways. Cdn Inst Food Sci Technol J 10(3):138.

Pugliese M, Lifshitz F, Fort D, Grad G, Marks-Katz M (1982). Fear of obesity - a new syndrome of delayed growth and sexual development in adolescence. Scientific paper presented at the 22nd Annual Meeting of the American Society for Clinical Nutrition, Washington DC, May.

Roberts LJ (1958). Beginnings of the recommended dietary allowances. J Am Dietet Assoc 34:903.

Sandstead HJ (1981). Methods for determining nutrient requirements in pregnancy. Am J Clin Nut 34:697.

Sweden. Swedish Food Regulations (1981). "Swedish Nutrition Recommendations", Uppsala: Swedish National Food Administration.

United States (1980). "Code of Federal Regulations 21 Food and Drugs Parts 100 to 169", Washington: Office of the Federal Register, National Archives and Records Service, General Services Administration.

USDA (United States Department of Agriculture) (1980). "Food and Nutrient Intakes of Individuals in 1 Day in the United States, Spring 1977", Washington: Science and Education Administration.

USDHEW (United States Department of Health, Education and Welfare) (1977). "Dietary Intake Findings, United States, 1971-1974", Hyattsville: National Center for Health Statistics.

Walker ARP, Walker BF (1981). Recommended dietary allowances and third world populations (editorial). Am J Clin Nutr 34:2319.

Watt BK (1980). Tables of food composition: uses and limitations. Contemporary Nutrition 5(2).

Young CM, Hagan GC, Tucker RE, Foster WD (1952). A comparison of dietary study methods II Dietary history vs. seven day record vs. 24-hour recall. J Am Dietet Assoc 28:218.

Diet, Nutrition, and Cancer:
From Basic Research to Policy Implications, pages 269–286
© *1983 Alan R. Liss, Inc., 150 Fifth Avenue, New York, NY 10011*

Traditional Education Approach: Does it Have Value?

Raymond E. Schucker, Ph.D.
Allan L. Forbes, M.D.
Bureau of Foods
Food and Drug Administration
Washington, DC 20204

As a scientific consensus begins to emerge regarding the role of diet in cancer, attention now turns to the implications for public policy and to a consideration of the means for its implementation. Given a national strategic objective of disease prevention in preference to less cost-effective remedial or palliative treatment, the potential of the education system as we know it for achieving cancer-related nutritional and dietary objectives must be carefully assessed. The assessment will need to go beyond the issue of knowledge transfer to the question of whether and in what ways traditional education should be augmented in order to achieve and sustain change in societal dietary habits.

Objectives for improved public knowledge of diet in relation to cancer and the other major degenerative diseases have been established by the Surgeon General. According to these objectives, a predominant majority of the American public by 1990 is to be able to identify the principal dietary factors involved in the diseases, and a majority of adults are to be able to identify the major foods that are low in fat, low in sodium, and high in calories, and foods that are good sources of fiber (U.S. Department of Health and Human Services 1980). More recently the National Academy of Sciences (NAS) in the report Diet, Nutrition and

Note: The views expressed in this paper are those of the authors and may not reflect those of the Food and Drug Administration or the Department of Health and Human Services in all respects.

<u>Cancer</u> (National Academy of Sciences 1982) has formulated
interim dietary guidelines that NAS considers consistent
with good nutritional practices and likely to reduce the
risk of cancer. The recommendations relating to diet are to:

o   reduce intake of saturated and unsaturated fats to
    30% of total calories in the diet

o   include fruits (especially citrus), vegetables
    (especially the dark green leafy and yellow
    vegetables) and whole grain cereal products in the
    daily diet

o   minimize consumption of food preserved by salt-
    curing or smoking

o   avoid excessive consumption of alcoholic beverages
    in combination with cigarette smoking.

With the one exception pertaining to fruits and
vegetables, the NAS guidelines advocate avoidance behavior
and call for rather profound changes affecting some of the
most deeply rooted hedonistic aspects of food and eating.
As will be reviewed, the evidence would suggest that the
role and techniques of education should be greatly expanded
around the concepts of behavior modification, self-management, and life style intervention. This paper surveys
recent progress in health-related behavior modification in a
general way and accomplishments in dietary behavior change
specifically. A great deal of research has involved dietary
intervention to reduce risk of heart disease. It is suggested that aspects of the diet-heart experience may serve
as a useful starting model for developing diet-cancer
education, both from the standpoint of setting achievable
objectives and as a source of techniques.

IN-SCHOOL NUTRITION EDUCATION

By and large, nutrition education in schools, i.e.,
the "bulk" of the traditional education approach, is still
deficiency-disease oriented, with emphasis placed on the
importance of consuming a variety of foods to ensure an
adequate intake of necessary nutrients. Only recently has
the emphasis in curriculum development turned to disease
prevention. Research on the effectiveness of primary and

secondary nutrition education has been characterized by mixed results. Available studies usually show strong impact of classroom instruction on factual knowledge. However, there are fewer instances in the literature of attitude change and only infrequent cases in which even short-term changes have been observed in behavioral measures such as cafeteria food selection, plate waste, and content of school lunch bags (Coates, et al 1981; Blakeway, Knickrehm 1978; Goldberg, et al 1980). That conventional school education has been more successful in imparting knowledge than in influencing dietary behavior was concluded in a recent large-scale evaluation of the National Nutrition Education and Training Program (NET) that reaches 3.4 million K-6 students under grants for the training of educators and food service personnel (St. Pierre, Rezmovic 1982). The philosophy of NET has been based in part on a cognitive theory which holds that the motivating force that changes attitudes, beliefs, and ultimately behavior is embedded in the process of learning new information.

Large-scale national surveys of food consumption show little indication that dietary habits have been influenced by traditional education over the last 20 years. The most striking changes in the population have been a reduction in caloric intake, shifts in consumption from higher fat to lower fat dairy products, and increased consumption of vegetable in relation to animal fat, avoidance behaviors that have not been the subject matter of nutrition education in public schools until very recently (Rizek, Jackson 1980; Enig, et al 1978).

Behavioral scientists are remarkably in agreement that a major weakness of formal nutrition education and other attempts at dietary information transfer is the failure to provide the individual with the necessary motivation to change behavior (Barlow, Tillotson 1978; Evans, Hall 1978; Mahoney, Caggiula 1978; Hochbaum 1981; Jacoby, et al 1981). Other reasons have been advanced for the lack of educational impact on national dietary habits. Classroom education programs have not been sustained for long enough periods of time during the formative years. Efforts have been spotty and for the most part confined to the primary grades. Classroom nutrition instruction touches only a very narrow aspect of living. It is not integrated with other facets of home, work, and social life.

In 1980 a national conference under the sponsorship of the Department of Health and Human Services (DHHS) met to assess the current status of nutrition education and needs for the future. A task force on the needs of the general public concluded that the traditional methods of formal education need to be bolstered and that dietary change must be sought in the home and community as well as in clinics and schools (Brown, Cooke 1980). Two components that are needed in the expanded effort include the broadcast media (both radio and television) and application of the principles and methods of social psychology, particularly those emerging from individual counseling and interventions to change unhealthy life style practices such as smoking, drug abuse, and overeating related to obesity.

DIETARY INTERVENTION AS A COMPONENT OF HEART DISEASE RISK PREVENTION TRIALS

The risk factors associated with coronary heart disease (CHD) have been extensively investigated for more than 30 years. Serum cholesterol and saturated fat intakes were early implicated in CHD through epidemiological studies, and the universality of the association was demonstrated by Keys and his co-workers in the well-known seven countries study (Keys, et al 1966). Experimental alteration of dietary fats and cholesterol among institutionalized volunteers demonstrated that serum cholesterol concentrations could be reduced. This gave impetus to larger scale studies of diet modification among free living populations. The results of this stream of research in diet intervention are of some relevance in approaching diet-cancer education, especially with respect to implementing the NAS guidelines for total dietary fat.

The first group of intervention studies to be reviewed were similar in some of their characteristics. Often there was concurrent intervention affecting more than one heart disease risk factor such as obesity, hypertension, and cigarette smoking, as well as diet. Specific dietary objectives were usually aimed at reducing cholesterol and saturated fat intakes. Reduction in total dietary fat was less often emphasized as a desirable end in itself, but in some programs was set as a secondary objective for weight control or to promote change to use of specific foods on recommended lists. Dietary training was usually administered in a combination of initial small group lecture and demonstration sessions, followed by periodic individual counseling. Participants were typically noninstitution-alized, middle-aged males at risk on the basis of one or more factors for heart disease and who had been informed about their risks at the outset.

In a study of myocardial infarct patients and their families who received continual diet supervision for eight years, Morrison (1955) reported an average serum cholesterol reduction of 29% at third year followup. The Anti-Coronary Club Program provided supervised adherence to a "prudent diet" for a group of participants on a monthly basis for six years. Average cholesterol reduction relative to a control group was 11%. The treatment group also achieved improvement in polyunsaturated fat in the diet as indicated by increasing levels of linoleic acid in analysis of depot fat (Christakis, et al 1966; Singman, et al 1980). In the two-year National Diet Heart Study, experimental groups given only instruction in how to maintain a dietary plan aimed at reducing serum cholesterol achieved cholesterol decreases of the same magnitude (12%) as other experimental groups that were provided blinded diets structured to lower total dietary fat and saturated fat (Brown 1968).

Similar results have been reported in Norway, Finland and Belgium by investigators who have used dietary interventions for extended periods of time to lower serum cholesterol and in some instances reduce reported consumption of total dietary fat (Leren 1970; Karvetti 1981; Kornitzer, et al 1980; Hjermann, et al 1981). Partially successful attempts to change dietary behavior have been reported in Sweden and Britain, in which dietary education efforts were not as intensive or were not sustained throughout the trial (Rose, et al 1980; Isaksson 1978). A conservative observation based on a recent review of the literature on clinical trials is that dietary intervention efforts on the whole have been equally as effective as the drug-assisted trials in achieving long-term serum cholesterol lowering (Rifkind, et al 1982).

Multiple Risk Factor Intervention Trial (MRFIT)

One of the largest clinical programs on heart disease prevention has been MRFIT. The objective was to undertake simultaneous intervention to reduce serum cholesterol, blood pressure, and cigarette smoking among men at the upper 10% level of risk but with no previous history of CHD (Zukel, et al 1981). A significant aspect of the trial compared with the other trials reported in this section was the substantial involvement of behavioral scientists in the design of the intervention components and in directing intervention activities at the 22 participating clinical centers during the six-year study.

The model for intervention drew heavily on social learning theory (Coates 1981; Bandura 1971; Maccoby, Farquhar 1975), concepts of behavioral self-management, and an array of guidance and behavioral modification techniques that were emerging from treatment programs for risk-taking behaviors such as overeating in obesity, smoking, drug abuse, and failure to adhere to prescribed drug use (McAlister, et al 1976; Dunbar, Stunkard 1979). A fundamental influence of the behavioral science input to MRFIT was to reorient intervention thinking away from the "medical model", i.e., the concept of the passive patient dependent on physician and nutritionist for guidance, to a view of the individual as an active participant in the process of setting his own goals and managing his own behavior toward achieving a given set of goals. The philosophy and design of the intervention have been reported in detail by Benfari (1981). The initial intervention was to consist of 10 group sessions attended by participant and spouse, supplemented by individual counseling. Extended intervention was on a one-to-one basis. Participants were instructed via an "eating pattern" approach rather than a prescribed diet (Sherwin, et al 1981).

In the first year a statistically significant mean serum cholesterol reduction of 6.3% was obtained in the dietary intervention group. The reduction held through four years among participants who regularly visited the clinic (Caggiula, et al 1981).

A secondary objective for total fat to be $\leq$ 35% of calories had initially been set to help reduce caloric intake for those needing to reduce weight and to fit the fat composition of the foods to be recommended to meet goals for saturated and unsaturated fat. At three years the intervention group had reduced fat to 33.8% of calories, and had achieved the reduction within the first year after intervention started. No change in fat consumption occurred in the control group (Neaton, et al 1981).

COMMUNITY INTERVENTION STUDIES

The dietary interventions of the clinical trials have consisted of fairly intensive personal education efforts among volunteers motivated in varying degrees by knowledge that they were at risk or as a result of having experienced coronary incidents. Two large-scale trials have been conducted under different conditions. Both studies had dietary intervention components aimed at risk reduction in the community as a whole and placed greater emphasis on use of the mass media to inform and instruct lower-risk participants.

The North Karelia Project

In the early 1970's elected officials in the county of North Karelia, Finland petitioned the national government for assistance in reducing morbidity and mortality rates from cardiovascular disease (CVD). Disease rates in the area were known to be among the highest in the country, and Finland had the highest incidence of CVD in the world. The intermediate objectives of the project were to reduce smoking, serum cholesterol, and blood pressure in the general population aged 30-59. To be included was an evaluation of the effects, costs, and other consequences of the program and an assessment of the feasibility of implementing a program nationally.

The principles and methods of intervention employed were premised on the use of the existing service structure and social organizations of the community. Baseline surveys conducted in North Karelia established that awareness and knowledge of the risk factors in CVD were already high among county inhabitants and that many attempts were being made individually to reduce risk. Consequently, the major project strategy was to create a spirit of joint effort, teach practical skills, develop social support and the environments to help people maintain changes, and to provide feedback about the community's achievements. Increased health knowledge was only a secondary goal. General information about the practical measures to be used against the risk factors was supplied by means of the mass media, health education material, and community meetings. Lay volunteers as well as health personnel were trained in program tasks. In comparison with a control county not receiving intervention, at the end of five years North Karelia male survey participants had statistically significant reductions of 4% in serum cholesterol, 13% in smoking, and 3% in systolic and diastolic blood pressure. Differences were less pronounced among women for smoking and cholesterol (Salonen, Puska, et al 1981). Although changes in the individual risk factors were small, taken in combination the gains produced an estimated 17% reduction among men in overall risk of CHD (Puska, et al 1979).

Further analysis of the data showed that health behavior changes were not consistently related to pre-intervention risk levels. It was concluded that health behavior change in the intervention community was based on common life style changes, and that either face-to-face counseling or new techniques of mass communication would be needed to induce high-risk individuals to make greater efforts to change their risk-related behaviors (Salonen, Heinonen, et al 1981). It was also shown that, while risk behaviors changed in the intervention community, already high knowledge levels did not further improve, indicating the validity of the strategy to support efforts already under way (Puska, et al 1981).

The Stanford Community Studies

At about the same time the North Karelia project got under way in Finland, a community study was undertaken in three small towns in the United States under the auspices of the Stanford Heart Disease Prevention Program. The objective was to determine whether mass media could be used as the primary mode of instruction in reducing the risk factors for heart disease among 35-59-year-old men and women. The dietary change component of the intervention focused principally on reducing consumption of cholesterol and saturated fats. Other goals were to reduce smoking and weight gain and to increase physical activity.

The design of the intervention was grounded in social learning theory and the dynamics of interpersonal and group processes. These have been extensively described (Maccoby, Farquhar, et al 1977; Maccoby, Solomon 1981), including the specific roles of television and radio as they were seen to fit into a behavior modification framework. One town was designated to receive mass media instruction only, a second town received mass media plus intensive face-to-face instruction for participants who were at high risk, and a third town served as a control.

Multiple media sources used in addition to television and radio were posters, billboards, newspaper medical columns, and direct mail. The media effort consisted of three hours of TV programming, several hours of radio programming, and multiple monthly airings of a rotating pool of 50 TV spots and 100 radio spots during the two-year campaign. A school kit consisting of heart-health materials was made available for teacher use in the 5th, 6th, and 7th grades.

Media development was a joint effort of specialists in behavioral sciences, mass communications and media production, and cardiovascular epidemiology. Mini-surveys were taken initially in the intervention communities to establish knowledge of heart disease risks and attitudes toward modifying risk behavior. Media materials were structured accordingly and key concepts and terminology were pretested for comprehension and communication effectiveness before incorporation into the campaign.

The media campaign lasted for two years, but at a reduced level of effort in year two in both intervention communities. High-risk participants in the single involved community additionally received 10 weeks of face-to-face instruction in small groups or in the form of at-home visits by counselors.

At the end of the second year, statistically significant reductions in dietary cholesterol and saturated fat consumption were reported in the intervention communities, with participants in the mass media-only town achieving about the same reductions as the town receiving media plus intensive instruction. There was a high correlation between change in reported dietary cholesterol and change in plasma cholesterol (Stern, et al 1976). Risk factor knowledge improvement and smoking reduction were somewhat better in the intensive instruction community at the end of the first year, but there were further substantial gains in the media-only town in the second year. As estimated by a multiple logistic risk function, overall risk reduction from all factors combined was equal across the two intervention communities, averaging 23% to 28% relative to control (Farquhar, et al 1977).   Plasma cholesterol differences continued to favor the two intervention towns over the control town in the third year, during which there were no media or instructional efforts (Fortmann, et al 1981).

An assessment of the overall outcome of the three-community study concluded that mass media increased knowledge and influenced behavior more readily in matters of diet than in the more refractive behaviors associated with overweight and smoking.   The need was identified to discover how the media can be used to stimulate and coordinate programs of interpersonal instruction in natural community groups, such as the worksite, and as a means to deliver special training and counseling regarding difficult behaviors such as smoking (Maccoby, Solomon 1981).

Other Community Interventions

A second project of the Stanford Heart Disease Prevention Program is now under way in five larger California cities.   These have more complex social structures which may offer more opportunities to facilitate change.   The study will last five to eight years and is targeted at the broader age range of 12 through 73 years. Greater attention is being paid to the in-school component of the program, which, due to limited resources, could not be fully developed in the original three-community study. Also, special emphasis is being given to fostering community education efforts that can maintain themselves indefinitely.   Outside involvement is being limited to development of the organizational plan, design and production of mass media materials, and the training of community volunteers who in turn will be responsible for coordinating all face-to-face instruction and other community action through local groups.

Interest in community-wide education for heart disease prevention continues to grow, and projects have now been started in Minnesota; Rhode Island; Lycoming County in Pennsylvania; New South Wales, Australia; South Africa; and Heidelberg, Germany.

ENVIRONMENT FOR DIET-CANCER EDUCATION

Some aspects of the climate in which the diet-cancer guidelines are emerging should be recognized in the development of dietary education programs. The first is the large gap between public perception of the seriousness of cancer among the major degenerative diseases and public belief that it may be diet related. Harris polls for the last decade have shown that well over 90% of adults consider cancer "very serious" for persons of their age, a slightly higher percentage than for CVD (Littleton, Boyd 1981). This may be contrasted with Food and Drug Administration (FDA) opinion surveys in 1978 and 1980 in which only about 20% of the lay public mentioned cancer when asked to name important diet-related health problems. In comparison, almost 50% mentioned heart disease as a health problem having a basis in diet. An FDA survey of food firms and members of the American Institute of Nutrition revealed substantially the same perceptions as those held by consumers (Heimbach, Stokes 1982).

Second, there is the serious problem of motivating people to change dietary habits when the health consequences of improper behavior may be far in the future. One of the major contributions of the behavioral sciences to diet-heart education has been to demonstrate that desirable interim target behaviors can be established and pursued by individuals in successive steps toward long term goals, and that successful performance of the behaviors, given proper reinforcement and social support, can provide the motivating force to keep the change process going. Important elements in the process are individual feedback and knowledge of results. Effective use can be made of biochemical measures such as serum cholesterol and triglycerides, weight loss data, carbon monoxide content of the breath, and blood pressure measures, for example, in providing the individual with knowledge of progress in reducing cholesterol and saturated fat intake, reducing calories, and cutting down smoking. With respect to the diet-cancer objectives, similar attention will need to be given to appropriate feedback indicators of change in total dietary fat and other interim dietary guidelines, which have received less emphasis in diet-heart education as desirable objectives in and of themselves.

A third issue is whether diet-heart and diet-cancer

education efforts should proceed independently or now be integrated, given the apparent convergence on the role of dietary fat in both diseases. With separate programs there is a major potential for confusing the public with overlapping and competing messages. It is reasonable to examine the other dietary parallels that might exist between approaches to CVD and cancer prevention, e.g., reduction in sodium intakes (for totally different reasons), as well as increments in certain fibrous materials from plant derived foods. A combined effort might offer the opportunity to achieve multiple health goals with the same set of dietary objectives. Another reason for considering the consolidation of certain aspects of heart and cancer education is to avoid raising unwarranted fears about the food supply, the seeds of which are already present in the negative emotional valence that attaches to cancer and which may underlie the current level of public concern about food additives, for example.

Fourth, the food industry is a contributing change agent in modifying food selection and eating habits over the long run. The marked increase in this country in consumption of vegetable oils and fats relative to animal fat over the last 20 (Enig, et al 1978) has been due in part to the ability of food processors to develop and market acceptable products containing less or no cholesterol and less saturated fats. For producers in the mainstream of the food supply this has largely been a technical and economic matter of substituting one fat for another without changing level of use, excluding those manufacturers of mostly dairy-based products who chose to market reduced fat products promoted as being lower in calories. For manufacturers not electing to market lower calorie products by reducing fat, yet who will be desirous of meeting consumer needs for foods that are directionally in line with the cancer guidelines, technology has yet to develop fats and oils substitutes that produce foods with the same sensory and satiating characteristics as their full fat counterparts. At least one promising constituent, polyester sucrose, is under investigation, but how soon it will become available commercially and the extent of its use as a replacement are unknown.

The food industy is becoming more active in seeking to reduce the sodium content of processed foods, exploring sodium substitutes, and making compensatory use of herbs and

spices in lieu of salt for flavoring purposes. Some progress is reported in modifying traditional salt-based preser-
vation processes. For example, pickles lower in sodium are
now entering the market. However, the prevailing opinion is
that dramatic breakthroughs with salt substitutes are not on
the immediate horizon and that consumer palates will need to
be re-educated to accept lower levels of salt in processed
foods.

ROLE OF THE FOOD LABEL

Brief mention should be made of the current status of
nutrition labeling in relation to the diet-cancer guidelines. The food label can assist shoppers in making better
informed food selections, given knowledge, the necessary
motivation, and the skills to use such information. Although a relatively passive component of the total education
process as envisioned in this discussion, the label is the
most widely available food information transfer system.

On a retail sales basis, over 40% of processed foods
now bear a declaration of total fat in grams per serving as
part of nutrition labeling. Fatty acids and cholesterol are
declared on 6% of foods. According to FDA research, among
shoppers who pay attention to the nutrition label, 20% say
fat content is the element most useful to them, mostly for
reasons related to calorie control (Heimbach, Stokes 1979).
Fat information could be aligned more closely with the
dietary guidelines by adding a declaration of percent of fat
from total calories. Greater prominence on the label could
be given to fat as well as other selected nutrient information through typography, and use of color and other
elements of format. Further guidance in enhancing specific
items of nutrition information will be forthcoming from a
project FDA is currently conducting to revise and simplify
the nutrition label so that it can be readily understood and
used by more consumers, particularly the undereducated and
those with diet-related health problems in the family.

Related less directly to the guideline on salt-
preserved food is the current voluntary initiative of the
DHHS and the food industry to provide quantitative sodium
labeling on more products in conjunction with efforts to
lower sodium levels in foods currently on the market. This
initiative has resulted in rapid growth in quantitative

sodium labeling, now available on about 13% of the food supply and expected at least to double within a year. FDA has also published a proposed regulation which would add a quantitative sodium declaration in milligrams per serving to all nutrition-labeled foods and would define terms such as "low sodium," "reduced sodium," and "sodium free."

DISCUSSION AND CONCLUSIONS

A compelling case for mass education has been made by Rose (1981) in calling attention to the "prevention paradox" in heart disease. This arises from the observation that the aggregate health benefit resulting from a small reduction in risk by many in the population can be as great as the achievement of a large reduction in risk among the relative-ly few who are at the upper end of the risk distribution. The paradox in Rose's view is that rational appeals to lower-risk individuals to modify their behavior will not be heeded because the individual will perceive his payoff to be small. Rose's recommendation is to use mass education to bring social pressure to bear to force change. We agree with the objective of mass education, but not in the pre-scribed application. The evidence from the better managed community-wide intervention studies clearly indicates that adults are in fact receptive to multi-source education inputs designed to impart knowledge of risk and to develop and reinforce skills for modifying risk-related behavior. Furthermore, among the risk factors in heart disease that have been targeted for education, dietary behavior has been relatively more responsive to mass media instruction and less dependent on face-to-face counseling than smoking, weight control and exercise behaviors.

Although the behavioral changes obtained in community-level programs have been small and the associated reductions in disease risk factors smaller still, their combined syner-gistic effects in reducing risk of CHD have been of practi-cal significance. The community approach has potential for diet-cancer education, perhaps integrated in some aspects with diet-heart education. Particular attention should first be given to raising the current low level of public knowledge of the diet-cancer risk relationship. Subsequent dietary behavior modification efforts should develop feedback measures of progress that can be used at the indi-vidual level to motivate and reinforce changes in dietary practices, particularly as they relate to total dietary fat.

To return to the question posed as the theme of this paper, we have suggested that formal education alone will not lead people to change their dietary practices. Minimally, the objectives of education must be reoriented from teaching facts on a deficiency disease basis to developing skills and training in avoidance behavior. The domain of education needs to be extended from the individual in the classroom to the family in the community. The mass media, particularly the broadcast media, should be adapted as teaching aids. Lastly, both the formal and informal components of community education should be continuous and capable of being sustained over time.

REFERENCES

Bandura A (1971). "Social Learning Theory." Morristown: General Learning Press.

Barlow DH, Tillotson JL (1978). Behavioral science and nutrition: a new perspective. J Am Diet Assoc 72:368-371.

Benfari RC (1981). The Multiple Risk Factor Intervention Trial (MRFIT) III: the model for intervention. Prev Med 10:426-442.

Blakeway SF, Knickrehm ME (1978). Nutrition education in the Little Rock School Lunch Program. J Am Diet Assoc 72:389-391.

Brown HB (1968). The National Diet-Heart Study - implications for dietitians and nutritionists. J Am Diet Assoc 52:279-287.

Brown KH, Cooke TM (1980). The general public: task force report to National Conference on Nutrition Education. J Nutr Educ 12(Suppl 1):117-120.

Caggiula AW, Christakis G, Farrand M, Hulley SB, Johnson R, Lasser NL, et al (1981). The Multiple Risk Factor Intervention Trial (MRFIT) IV: intervention on blood lipids. Prev Med 10:443-476.

Christakis G, Rinzler SH, Archer M, Kraus A (1966). Effect of the Anti-Coronary Club Program on coronary heart disease risk factor status. J Am Med Assoc 198:597-604.

Coates TJ (1981). New strategies for changing dietary behavior. In Hefferen JJ, Ayer WA, Koehler HM (eds): "Foods, Nutrition and Dental Health," Park Forest South: Pathotox, pp 191-206.

Coates TJ, Jeffery RW, Slinkard LA (1981). Heart healthy eating and exercise: introducing and maintaining changes in health behaviors. Am J Public Health 1:15-23.

Dunbar JM, Stunkard AJ (1979). Adherence to diet and drug regimen. In Levy R, Rifkind B, Dennis B, Ernst N (eds): "Nutrition, Lipids and Coronary Heart Disease," New York: Raven, pp 391-423.

Enig MG, Munn RJ, Keeney M (1978). Dietary fat and cancer trends - a critique. Fed Proc 9:2216-2220.

Evans RI, Hall Y (1978). Social-psychologic perspective in motivating changes in eating behavior." J Am Diet Assoc 72:378-383.

Farquhar JW, Maccoby N, Wood PD, Alexander JK, Breitrose H, Brown Jr BW, et al (1977). Community education for cardiovascular health. Lancet 1:1192-1195.

Fortmann SP, Williams PT, Hulley SB, Haskell WL, Farquhar JW (1981). Effect of health education on dietary behavior: The Stanford Three Community Study. Am J Clin Nutr 34:2030-2038.

Goldberg SJ, Allen HD, Friedman G, Meredith K, Tymrack M, Owen AY (1980). Use of health education and attempted dietary change to modify atherosclerotic risk factors: a controlled trial. Am J Clin Nutr 6:1272-1278.

Heimbach JT, Stokes RC (1982). "Nutrition Labeling for Today's Needs: Opinions of Nutritionists, the Food Industry, and Consumers." Washington: Food and Drug Administration.

Heimbach JT, Stokes RC (1979). "FDA 1978 Consumer Food Labeling Survey." Washington: Food and Drug Administration.

Hjermann I, Byre KV, Holme I, Leren P (1981). Effect of diet and smoking intervention on the incidence of coronary heart disease. Lancet 2:1303-1310.

Hochbaum GM (1981). Strategies and their rationale for changing people's eating habits. J Nutr Educ 13(Supp 1): 59-65.

Isaksson B (1978). The Swedish Diet and Exercise Program. BNF Nutr Bul 4:228-233.

Jacoby J, Olson JC, Szybillo GJ, Hart EW (1981). Behavioral science perspectives on conveying nutrition information to consumers. In Solms J, Hall RL (eds): "Criteria of Food Acceptance: How Man Chooses What He Eats," Zurich: Foster, pp 13-25.

Karvetti RL (1981). Effects of nutrition education. J Am Diet Assoc 79:660-667.

Keys A, Aravanis C, Blackburn HW, Van Buchem FSP, Buzina R, Djordjevic BS, et al (1966). Epidemiological studies related to coronary heart disease: characteristics of men aged 40-59 in seven countries. Acta Med Scand 460(Suppl): 1-392.

Kornitzer M, De Backer GD, Dramaix M, Thilly C (1980). The Belgian Heart Disease Prevention Project: modification of the coronary risk profile in an industrial population. Circulation 61:18-25.

Leren P (1970). Oslo Diet-Heart Study 11-year report. Circulation 42:935-942.

Littleton AC, Boyd MW (1981). "The Public and High Blood Pressure." Washington: National Institutes of Health, No 81-2118.

McAlister BA, Farquhar JW, Thoresen CE, Maccoby N (1976). Behavioral science applied to cardiovascular health: progress and research needs in the modification of risk-taking habits in adult populations. Health Educ Monogr 4:45-74.

Maccoby N, Farquhar JW (1975). Communication for health: unselling heart disease. J Commun 25:114-126.

Maccoby N, Farquhar JW, Wood PD, Alexander, MA (1977). Reducing the risk of cardiovascular disease: effects of a community-based campaign on knowledge and behavior. J Comm Health 3:100-114.

Maccoby N, Solomon D (1981). The Stanford Community Studies in heart disease prevention. In Rice R, Paisley W (eds): "Public Communication Campaigns," Beverly Hills: Sage.

Mahoney MJ, Caggiula AW (1978). Applying behavioral methods to nutritional counseling. J Am Diet Assoc 72:372-377.

Morrison IM (1955). A nutritional program for prolongation of life in coronary atherosclerosis. J Am Med Assoc 159:1425-1428.

National Academy of Sciences (1982). "Diet, Nutrition and Cancer." Washington: National Academy Press.

Neaton JD, Broste S, Cohen L, Fishman EL, Kjelsberg MO, Schoenberger J (1981). The Multiple Risk Factor Intervention Trial (MRFIT) VII: a comparison of risk factor changes between the two study groups. Prev Med 10:519-544.

Puska P, Tuomilehto J, Salonen JT, Neittaanmaki L, Maki J, Virtamo J, et al (1979). Changes in coronary risk factors during comprehensive five-year community programme to control cardiovascular diseases during 1972-1977 in North Karelia. Br Med J 2:1173-1178.

Puska P, Vienola P, Kottke TE, Salonen JT, Neittaanmaki L (1981). Health knowledge and community prevention of coronary heart disease. Int J Health Educ 24(Supp 2):1-11.

Rifkind BM, Goor R, Schucker B (1982). Compliance and cholesterol lowering in clinical trials: efficacy of diet. To be published in the Proceedings of the 6th International Symposium on Atherosclerosis, Berlin, West Germany.

Rizek RL, Jackson EM (1980). "Current Food Consumption Practices and Nutrient Sources in the American Diet." Washington: Consumer Nutrition Center, Science and Education Administration, U.S. Department of Agriculture.

Rose G (1981). Strategy of prevention: lessons from cardiovascular disease. Br Med J 282:1847-1851.

Rose G, Heller RF, Pedoe HT, Christi DGS (1980). Heart Disease Prevention Project: a randomised controlled trial in industry. Br Med J 280:747-751.

St. Pierre RG, Rezmovic V (1982). An overview of the national nutrition education and training program evaluation. J Nutr Educ 14:61-66.

Salonen JT, Heinonen OP, Kottke TE, Puska P (1981). Change in health behavior in relation to estimated coronary heart disease risk during a community-based cardiovascular disease prevention programme. Int J Epidemiol 4:343-354.

Salonen JT, Puska P, Kottke TE, Tuomilehto J (1981). Changes in smoking, serum cholesterol and blood pressure levels during a community-based cardiovascular disease prevention program - The North Karelia Project. Am J Epidemiol 114:81-94.

Sherwin R, Kaelber CT, Kezdi P, Kjelsberg MO, Thomas Jr HE (1981). The Multiple Risk Factor Intervention Trial (MRFIT) II: the development of the protocol. Prev Med 10:402-426.

Singman HS, Berman SN, Cowell C, Maslansky E, Archer M (1980). The Anti-Coronary Club: 1957 to 1972. Am J Clin Nutr 33:1183-1191.

Stern MP, Farquhar JW, Maccoby N, Russell SH (1976). Results of a two-year health education campaign on dietary behavior: The Stanford Three Community Study. Circulation 54:826-833.

U.S. Department of Health and Human Services (1980). "Promoting Health and Preventing Disease." Washington: U.S. Government Printing Office.

Zukel WJ, Oglesby P, Schnaper HW (1981). The Multiple Risk Factor Intervention Trial (MRFIT) I: historical prespectives. Prev Med 10:387-402.

Index

Acetylaminofluorene, 11
Acinar cell nodules of pancreas, 35
  dietary fats affecting, 41
  predictive nature of, 41–42, 43
  quantitation of, 41–42
Adenocarcinoma
  mammary gland. *See* Mammary
    gland cancer
  pancreatic. *See* Pancreatic cancer
Aflatoxin, 144, 145
  epidemiology of cancer risk from,
    157
Aflatoxin B_1
  cancer risk assessment of, 161–162,
    163
  carcinogenicity of, 155
    relative to other aflatoxins, 160,
      161
    testing of, 157
  hepatic, 155
Aflatoxin M_1
  cancer risk assessment of, 161–162,
    163
  human exposure to, 161
  relative carcinogenicity of, 160, 161
Alcohol consumption and cancer,
  270
Alkaloids, pyrrolizidine, 204
Alkylating agents in tumorigenesis, 9
Ames/*Salmonella* mutagenicity test,
  159
  of cooked meat, 180
  foodborne carcinogens detection by,
  204

Anticarcinogenic agents
  in food, 141–152
  protease inhibitors, 167–174
Antigenotoxic agents, identification of
  body fluid effect on, 145–148
  in foods, 141–152
  saliva affecting, 145–148
  test development for, 148–152
  in vitro assays for, 141–145
Antioxidants
  vs dietary fats in carcinogenesis, 61,
    62, 63
    of mammary gland, 64, 66–68
  in mammary gland development, 80
  in photocarcinogenesis, 54–56
Asbestos, 222, 225
Ascorbic acid in photocarcinogenesis,
  85
Aspergillus in mycotoxin production,
  155, 156
Azaserine
  action of, 34
  pancreatic cancer induction by, 33–
    45

B

Bacillus subtilis, 156
Beans, 187
Beef
  in colon cancer etiology, 246
  mutagens in, 177–190
Benzoyl peroxide, 169
  in skin cancer, 63
Betel quid, 149, 151